Copyright 2018 Cassandra Allen
All rights reserved
Published by Cassandra Allen/Lulu Press, Inc.
627 Davis Drive, Suite 300, Morrisville, NC 27560

Scripture quotations marked KJV are from the Holy Bible,
King James Version
(Authorized Version) First published in 1611, Quoted from
the KJV Classic Copyright Reference Bible,
Copyright 1983 by Zondervan Corporation.

Scripture quotations marked NLT are taken from the Holy
Bible, New Living Translation,
Copyright 1996, 2004 and 2007

ISBN 978-0-578-20887-9

SPECIAL ACKNOWLEDGEMENTS

I give God all the glory for delivering me and giving me such a powerful testimony to share with the world. He is truly the head of my life.

A special thanks to Reverend Nancy Doolittle who I spoke with on the phone at my job but I've never met in person. Thank you for all your prayers and encouraging words. Thank you for all that you taught me during our time together. You tried to tell me that you didn't think God would leave us together much longer and then one day you were gone. I miss and love you so much.

Thank you to all the ladies in the prayer group who never stopped praying for me. Miss Grace, Miss Bernetta, Miss Ida, Sister Barbara, Sister Phyllis and Jolana I love you all to life.

A special acknowledgement to Mrs. Ida Clark who has always believed in every project I've worked on. Thank you for your support and financial blessings.

Thank you to my son Terry Peak, Jr. who held me accountable and encouraged me to finish this book.

613.8
ALL

**PROPERTY OF
EAST CHICAGO LIBRARY**

Growing up my life was filled with pain and struggles. I was in an abusive relationship for many years, but by the grace of God I got out alive. After that I suffered mental, verbal and emotional abuse. It seemed as though abuse was a normal way of life so I accepted and embraced it. I think maybe I was addicted to abuse as strange as it may sound.

There were so many things I didn't understand about myself. I didn't understand why my life had spiraled out of control. It seemed as though I would never recover from all the awful things that happened to me. I tried to figure things out on my own but I was only making it worse. I never thought for a second that I would survive all the turmoil in my life. I was puzzled for a long time as to why negative things kept happening to me. The harder I tried, the more hopeless it seemed. I was convinced that I was destined to live a life of destruction. It seemed as though good things were happening to everyone except me. I didn't understand why and I wanted things to change. I no longer wanted to carry the hurt, disappointment and pain that was buried deep inside of me. I had no answers to the questions running through my mind. I was always thinking, trying to figure out what went wrong and how I ended up in such a dark place. Perhaps I didn't want to remember because the pain would be too much for me to bare. I cried out to God hoping he would reveal the truth to me. I prayed and asked him to show me myself as he sees me. I knew it could be painful to relive the past, but I had to know who I really was. I had to know why my heart was broken into so many pieces.

    I wasn't raised in a church and I didn't have a relationship with God growing up. We went to church with my mother but I don't remember learning a lot. We learned songs and had speeches for Christmas and Easter. I may not remember much from back then but I do believe a foundation was laid for my life. We were taught the importance of family, friends and education. But we were not taught the importance of having God first in our lives. I wasted so much time chasing things that weren't really important at all. I was lost wanting worldly things instead of Godly things. Sometimes I wonder how my life would have turned out if I had spent it serving God. Sometimes I want to cry because I love the Lord with all my heart and soul and I want to please Him. I don't know the bible or all of the instructions in it but I hope one day that I will. I don't know God's plan for my life yet, but I'm grateful for the opportunity to have a relationship with Him. I will spend the rest of my life serving the Lord and seeking a closer relationship with

Him. I love the Lord with all my heart and nothing will ever separate me from Him again. I have broken several of God's commandments over and over again. I've lied, cheated, stolen and the list just goes on and on.

For some reason my mom and I have never really had a close relationship and I don't know why? My brother and sister say that we're just alike and maybe we are. I've always wanted to have a normal relationship with my mother but it hasn't happened yet. Sometimes I wonder if I should just stop trying but that's not an option. I know God can restore relationships so I'll keep praying and asking God for his divine intervention. It seems like our relationship changed when I was a teenager. My mother was convinced I was messing with boys but I wasn't and she called me some pretty nasty names. There was a short period of time that we did get along but I have very few memories of good times that we had together. I was the middle child and found it to be an uncomfortable place. When I wanted to do the things my brother did, I couldn't because he was older than me. When I asked to have the things my sister had I couldn't because she was younger than me. Somehow it just didn't seem fair. Living in the house with my mom and sister was especially difficult for me to face every day. The fact that they had a mother daughter relationship and we didn't was very hurtful. It wouldn't be as hard if I didn't live with them but I think God was telling me to stay there until He heals me of all the brokenness. The things my mother does still hurt so badly and I don't want it to hurt anymore. I pray and ask God to change me so that I'm more understanding of how she feels. I try to accept it, forgive it, forget it and not let it affect me but it still does. I asked God to forgive me for feeling this way but only He knows what's broken inside me. I try not to complain and I try to put on a happy face and fit in but the hurt and the pain inside are often overwhelming. There are days when I cry when it's time for me to go home. Some days I go to the store and look around just to delay going home. Other days I just sit in the parking lot at the grocery store and cry because it feels like I have no place to go. I know God is able to turn things around in an instant and I'll always believe that He will. I pray and ask God to strengthen me. I know God is still in control and He knows exactly how to fix me. I trust Him completely but I still lose my way sometimes. I try to focus on God through the good times and the bad because trouble won't last always. I pray that the Lord will teach me how to leave the past in the past and move forward. God says to ask and it shall be given so I'll just ask Him. God help me to forgive everyone who has hurt and abandoned me, just as you forgave me. God heal me of all the hurt, pain and bruises that are on the inside of me. Lord, I thank you for shielding me from my enemies. I know that you are working in and through me and I'll continue to give you the glory as you clean me up on the inside. I feel like my life had been ripped apart at the seams, but thank you Lord for putting me back together.

In the past few years I remembered that I was molested as a child. My memory is cloudy concerning the incident and I don't remember any details. There was some type of sexual interaction between myself and two male relatives who were both older than me. When it happened I was in elementary school because I do remember the house we lived in at the time. I don't think about it often but when I do I blame myself for allowing it to happen and I feel dirty and ashamed. One day it was on my mind and I told my mother what I could remember of it. I don't know what I wanted her to say but she didn't say anything and I couldn't understand that. Why didn't my mother care that I had been molested? I wanted her to talk to me about it. I wanted her to care that it happened to me but it didn't seem to interest her at all. I was confused and hurt that she didn't ask any questions about what happened. I used to wonder if I was cursed because of the things that happened in my childhood. Have I caused my children to be cursed too? I know now that Jesus has redeemed me from the curse of the law.

    I had my first boyfriend when I was seventeen. I got pregnant and was afraid to tell my parents. I pray every day and ask God to help me to forgive myself but I haven't been able to do that yet. Now that I'm closer to God and fear Him, I'm so afraid because of the things that I've done.

My whole life I lived in the same place and did the same things but I began to grow tired of this repetition and I wanted something different in my life. I wanted to change because I couldn't continue in the same way. I cried for so long asking God to help me and it didn't seem as if he ever would. I was smothering in my surroundings. I was on drugs and messing up my life and no one wanted to have anything to do with me. I was lost for so long but finally I was ready to do something different. I was convinced I couldn't accomplish this while living in the same place and being around the same people. Maybe it was guilt or shame because of how I looked or the things I had done but I knew I had to get away from it all. I couldn't concentrate on getting better and worry about what people were saying at the same time. The fact that no one in my family wanted anything to do with me didn't help either. Eventually, I moved away when I thought God was telling me I could go. I had been praying for a long time asking God to get me away from this place and He finally did. When I left I thought I would never come back but I did.

    When I moved away I had the opportunity to come closer to God. I thought I would be more patient with the troubles around me. Even though I had grown in the Lord and could see things more clearly I still had a long way to go. I know I still have a lot of stuff inside me that God is dealing with so I just continue to pray for deliverance. I know that God truly does answer prayers. I also know that He sees my tears that are constantly streaming down my face. He knows everything I'm going through and only He can deliver me. God allows us to go through things in order to grow in endurance and maturity. The devil will use whomever he can to carry out his evil deeds and not everyone can recognize this. Because my flesh gets in the way, I probably complicate things that I go through. I pray that God will see fit to deliver me from this thorn in my side. The enemy is trying to destroy me but I won't give up and I'm not afraid anymore. I must repent and be cleansed of all unrighteousness. I know I'm guilty of many sins and some of them are detestable but I know that God forgives. I know that Jesus Christ was crucified on the cross and resurrected on the third day and all my sins are forgiven. I know there are still hurt, pain and anger in my heart. They have become like a force that is weighing me down and I no longer want them there. I don't know how these seeds were planted inside of me but they must have taken root by now. I decree and declare that no weapon formed against me shall prosper. Something is trying to control me and cause me to do things I don't want to do. Suddenly I can see things now that I could never see before. My heart must be circumcised and cleansed of all unrighteousness. I don't know what it is but I can feel it inside me. I pray that God will have mercy on me and fix everything that's broken in me. I wish I had known that the answer was to give everything to God. Because when I finally gave it all to Him, He brought me through it. There was no way I could have made it without Him. Sometimes I break down and cry because I love the Lord with all my heart and soul. I want nothing more than to please Him in all that I do.

    My parents were married until the day my dad died and I saw a lot of things. My dad was an alcoholic for a large part of my childhood but when I was a teenager he went into recovery. Because of dad's alcoholism there was plenty of turmoil inside our house. I grew up in a dysfunctional household. There was fighting, yelling, name calling and cursing going on much of the time. My dad was never home a lot because he worked, drank and spent plenty of time outside our home. This left my mom alone to take care of my siblings and me. I can imagine this was very difficult for my mother. Eventually she started doing things to keep herself busy while he was away. I often wonder how this affected my life and some of the choices I've made.

While I was in high school I starting drinking and smoking weed. Prior to this I was an exceptional student but my grades began to slip. I started skipping school and losing interest in my studies. One day I went off school grounds at lunch time with a small group of friends. I thought we were going to smoke weed but someone had laced the marijuana joints with another drug. We were walking around the neighborhood passing joints back and forth, laughing and having a good time. Then suddenly I felt really strange. It seemed as though I was in a dream but I wasn't. Everything was going in slow motion all around me. When we made it back to the school I walked into the building and I thought everyone was staring at me. People were laughing and pointing at me or at least I thought they were. I tried to find my next class but I was lost and couldn't find my way. I bumped into someone who was in my class and he showed me the way. I sat there and as the teacher began to talk I started falling asleep. I couldn't hold my head up and it kept falling down banging against the desk. It was disruptive and the teacher asked me to leave the classroom. I wandered up and down the hallways in a fog until a male friend offered to walk me home. When I got home my brother was home and I got into bed and went to sleep. I'm glad my brother was there because I'm sure he had planned to take advantage of me sexually.

I wasn't really interested in boys at first but the minute I got a boyfriend I got pregnant right away. I was afraid to tell my parents and I had no idea what to do. It was my senior year in high school and I was in love with him. I thought he loved me too, but I found out that he had been cheating on me the entire time we had been together. My parents were disappointed in me and I was disappointed in myself. My mother told me that I could only live in the house until I had the baby and I couldn't come back after that. Later on in my pregnancy she told me that she changed her mind because I was too stupid to take care of a child by myself. I had never felt so alone in my entire life. I thought I could make him want to be with me and not the others girls but I was wrong. The harder I tried to be good enough for him, the more hurt and devastated I became. Unfortunately, now that I was pregnant everyone was telling me all the things he had been doing. I was crushed and heartbroken so I broke up with him. I came to the realization that he never deserved me anyway. Soon after our break up he enlisted in the military. I thought he did it for me and our unborn child but I was wrong. He already had another girl pregnant and he married her. I had lost my virginity and fell in love with a man who didn't love me back. After my son was born I began to date again and continued to make poor choices in men. I just wanted someone to love me but I was looking for love in all the wrong places.

    I was going to parties and putting myself in dangerous situations. One night I went to a club and a man who I didn't know asked me to ride to his house with him. I got into the car with a total stranger and rode off with him. I had just met him and didn't know anything about this man. I told him that I wouldn't go inside his house and I would wait in the car for him. When we got there he invited me inside and I said no. He tried using every excuse he could think of to get me inside but I still refused to go in. I thought if I went inside the house I may not get out so I stayed outside where I felt safer. I was quite a distance away from the club and it was late at night. He refused to take me back to the club until I went inside with him. I had no choice but to get out of the car and start walking. I didn't know the area too well and it was very dark outside. I started walking and I saw a familiar high school in the distance. I cut across the empty parking lot and walked to a friend's house. My friend took me back to the club and dropped me off. When I look back at this night I knew God was with me because I could have been raped or even killed. No one would have ever known who I had left the club with. I never did anything like that again.

My life as an addict began long ago. I grew up around alcohol and drugs. Addiction was coming at me from both sides of my family. It was a bullet that was hard for me to dodge. At family gatherings there was always someone drinking alcohol and smoking marijuana. There was always a fight amongst us because of the drinking and drugs. I was drinking before I finished high school and shortly after that I tried cocaine for the very first time. I remember that day very clearly. I was with my girlfriend and we went to the bathroom together. She pulled out a vial that had a tiny spoon attached. She told me this was cocaine and I watched her sniff the powder off the spoon. She asked me if I wanted to try it and I said yes. I don't know why I said yes because I didn't even know what it was. I only knew that she sold it and made a lot of money. She always drove nice cars and had nice things. I tried it but I didn't like the way it made me feel so I didn't use it again until several years later. Shortly after that I let her convince me to sell cocaine too. This way I could make money and have nice things just like she did. So she gave me the cocaine to sell and told me that I didn't have to pay her until I sold it. The problem was that I didn't know anybody who used it. I eventually gave it back to her and our friendship didn't last long after that. She went on to have a successful life and I went on to become an addict.

One day I went to the hair salon to schedule an appointment. I met a man outside and we exchanged phone numbers. It was a week or so before he called me and the conversation didn't go very well. We just didn't seem to have anything in common. Eventually, he called again and slowly we began to spend time together. I didn't think I would really get involved with him but I did. As it turned out we would be connected for the rest of our lives.

When my cousin found out that I was dating him she told me that he was physically abusive to his girlfriends. I didn't believe her because I hadn't seen any signs of anger or violence from him. He had never even raised his voice to me so far. I thought I finally had a decent man. He had a good job, a house and he had a daughter. One day I was at his house and we were supposed to be going out. He went upstairs and he told me he would be right back. I waited by the door for what seemed like forever but he never came back downstairs. I kept calling his name but he didn't answer. Finally I went upstairs and he was in his bedroom with the door closed. I pushed the door open and the first thing I saw was what I now know to be crack cocaine and drug paraphernalia. I turned and started back down the stairs racing to get out of the house. I didn't understand what I had just seen but I knew something wasn't right. He ran after me and caught me at the door. I should have left then but I stayed. Staying in places I know I shouldn't be in has been one of my biggest downfalls. I know now that whenever I think I should leave a place or a situation to leave immediately. Now that his secret was out, he became bolder with his drug use. He disappeared for days at a time binging. I wouldn't hear from him and I didn't know where he was or who he was with. Some days I got in my car and drove to his friends' houses to see if he was there. There were times that I went to his house and knocked on the door but he wouldn't answer. I could hear voices inside but he didn't let me in because they were getting high. One day he and I were visiting a friend of his when my cousin and her friend walked in. My boyfriend continued to ignore my attempts to contact him.

After a while I started hanging out with my cousin and her friend. I figured this way I would eventually run into him since they visited the same people. All of the places we went were either drug dealers or drug users. My cousin and her friend were getting high and I started snorting cocaine with them. I would meet up with them every night and we rode around for hours looking and stopping at different houses. I didn't know the men we were hanging around so I sat quietly while they talked to them and I got high. I guess I didn't mind the way the drugs made me feel this time because I kept on using. Eventually I started visiting these men alone.

I knew they wanted to have sex with me so I kept going to see them. They continued to give me drugs while attempting to entice me to prostitute myself. I never had sex with any of them because I didn't have to. I only had to flirt a little bit and tell them that I would have sex with them and they kept supplying me with cocaine. I know that God was with me even then because once again I could have been raped and/or killed. I was constantly playing games with these men and using them for their drugs. I thank God that He has never stopped loving me even through all my sin. Although I got plenty of drugs for free, they wouldn't fall for my tactics for long. In the beginning I was trying to catch my boyfriend there but in the process I was using more and more. At some point it wasn't even about my boyfriend anymore, it was all about drugs. I was going to get high and get attention from these men. My boyfriend's priority was getting high and I was starving for his attention. I thought by hanging out with these men he would get jealous and start spending time with me but that didn't work. I sat around talking to these men while they got high and eventually they would offer me some too. I was using more and they were talking about sex more. The conversation was so disrespectful and degrading but I kept coming around for the drugs. In my right mind I would have never allowed anyone to talk to me this way. I thought I was outsmarting them but I was only fooling myself. It really didn't matter what they said because I never thought I would sleep with any of them. They watched me transform and all the while they planned to have sex with me at their leisure. I was promising to do sexual favors if they got me high and once I was high I would make up an excuse why I had to leave. Once I told one of the men that I would have sex with him so he rented a hotel room. He had to rent the room because he didn't want my boyfriend to find us together. I never had any intention of having sex with him; I just wanted to keep getting high. He laid there waiting for me to have sex with him while we continued to get high. I kept telling him that if he gave me just a little more we could have sex. Eventually he realized I was lying and he went to sleep. I just sat there looking pitiful and desperate until he woke up and took me home.

It wasn't long after that my boyfriend started to beat me. It happened just like my cousin had warned me. He punched me with his fist and gave me a black eye which not only devastated and confused me but I was traumatized. I was ashamed because I had to go to my parents' house and face them. He apologized days later and I went right back to seeing him again. This was the beginning of many years of physical abuse at the hands of this man. He beat me so many times I couldn't begin to count them. He went to jail more than once for domestic violence against me but I always went right back to him. One time I even dropped the charges against him so he could get out of jail. My mind was so messed up that I was convinced that when he got out he would be sorry and never hit me again. This made no sense at all but I couldn't help the way that I was. Anytime we argued I was always afraid that he would beat me up and he always did. I couldn't wrap my mind around the fact that I was in an abusive relationship and I didn't leave him. He beat me on a regular basis and I had several black eyes and lots of cuts and bruises. There was a time that he hit me and both of my eyes turned black. He would beat me up and leave and then I laid around waiting for him to call me and come back to me. Everyone around us knew what was going on. The police knew and all of our family and friends knew what was happening. One day my son was with us and he locked me in the bedroom and beat me. My son was outside the door screaming and banging to get in but that didn't stop him from beating me. He even beat me in front of his own mother and no one could make him stop hitting me. Once we were riding in the car and he told me that he was going to beat me up when we got home. I was determined not to be beaten that day so I jumped out of the car at a red light and ran into a nearby gas station. They locked the door and called the police. There was another occasion when we were on our way home and he was threatening to beat me up again. This time he ran all the lights and stop signs so I couldn't get out of the car. That didn't stop me because I jumped out of the car while we were still moving. As a result of this my hip was pulled out of socket and I had to have it replaced. He called me stupid for jumping out but I felt lucky to be alive. There was another time that he saw me driving my car and tried to make me pull over to talk to him but I refused because of the look in his eyes. I knew it would not end well for me so I kept going. He continued to chase me on the highway demanding that I pull over but I wouldn't stop. I drove faster and so did he trying to force me off the road. Eventually, he crashed into a pole and totaled his sister's car. I was hysterical but I kept driving and screaming until I made it home. He called me on the phone and was even more upset with me because I didn't stop to see if he was alright after the crash. I was a complete mess both physically and mentally. I was very depressed and when I wasn't high I just sat around and cried a lot. Getting high seemed to numb the pain and I didn't have to think about what was going on. My family was telling me that I liked being beaten by him because I didn't leave. They didn't understand that I couldn't leave and what's worse is I didn't know why. I already knew how messed up I was and hearing others say it only made me feel worse. He told me how sorry he was and that it would never happen again but it always did. I was extremely damaged from the bad relationships and the physical and emotional abuse. This time I didn't stop using drugs because my life had spiraled out of control. I stayed in this relationship for more than five years and suffered some serious injuries that have lasted a lifetime. I've had a broken nose, broken hip, black eyes and countless scars some of which still remain today.

For a while I was a functioning addict who still worked and paid my bills. But the enemy was working overtime trying to destroy me. I thought snorting cocaine was fun even though my nose was always runny and sore. I thought I was in total control of everything I did but I couldn't see the real truth. Addiction was setting me up to take over every aspect of my life. I would have never made a lot of the choices I did if I wasn't on drugs. My performance on my job was terrible because I was using and being abused. I worked about twenty miles from home and sometimes I let my boyfriend drop me off at work. Some days he didn't even bother to pick me up because he was getting high. I was so desperate to be in a relationship and to be loved that I accepted all of his behaviors. I was going to work beaten, bruised and eyes blackened. Finally, my job sent me to be evaluated. I went to a hospital where I begged them to admit me because I was depressed and tired. I was diagnosed with major depression and stayed in the hospital for 28 days. I didn't know that they tested my blood for drugs when I was admitted. While I was there I talked a lot about the abuse but I never mentioned my drug use. They tried to get me to admit it but I wouldn't. It wasn't until I got out of the hospital that my parents told me that the hospital had known the entire time that I was using drugs.

With the therapy and professional help I had received I thought my head was clear and I was home free but I wasn't. Not long after I was released I was seeing the same man and of course the beatings continued. I was too ashamed to go back to my job after they had tried to help me so I quit. I got pregnant and had my second son. I didn't use drugs while I was pregnant but I wanted to. My boyfriend wouldn't let me and I knew it was for the best. Throughout my pregnancy he stole so much from me. He was staying out all night on a regular basis. He was using my car so I had no way to go out and search for him. It was hard for me to know he was getting high and I couldn't. I knew as soon as my child was born I was going to get high again. Throughout my pregnancy he continued to get high. Somedays he took me to my parent's house early in the morning on his way to work. He was supposed to come back and get me after work but often he didn't. One day he picked me up and I didn't feel well. We were living with his sister at the time. We went home and he tucked me in bed and said he wanted to go to the liquor store. I was okay with that but I asked him to hurry back because I thought I was in labor. I fell asleep and when the alarm rang the next morning he wasn't in bed with me. I stood up to shut off the alarm and my water broke. No one had seen or heard from him so his sister dropped me off at the hospital on her way to work. I was too ashamed to call my parents so I gave birth all alone. It wasn't until the next day that he showed up at the hospital. I was angry and hurt and I didn't want to see him. I took one look at him and I knew he had been getting high. I forgave him again because I didn't have a choice and when I was released from the hospital the three of us went back home. He continued to go out and get high and not come home. I had reached my limit with him so I packed my things and our son and went back to my parent's house. I was so lost and I felt like the only thing I could do was get high. Addiction was living in me and controlling me. I had two kids by two different men yet I was still alone. My children were supposed to have the same father and I was supposed to have a husband. Getting high was all I had left. I was embarrassed to really go around my friends because no one had messed up like I had. If I just kept to myself and got high I wouldn't have to face anyone or talk to anyone. That was a very lonely place but what choice did I have. This was my life now and I had to live it.

I got a place of my own for my children and me. We lived in a small two bedroom house and things were going pretty good. I was working and had one child in school and the other one in daycare. I starting dating again but I never stopped using drugs. There was a man who lived next door and he was married. One day I came home from work and he had put a note in my mailbox. He was asking if I would go out with him and I foolishly accepted the invitation. We talked on the phone all the time and even went out to dinner a couple of times. Once we went on vacation to Indianapolis together because he was in a golf tournament. Eventually he began to spend the night at my house and his wife found out about us. When I think of all the wrong I've done, the people I've hurt and the lives I've ruined I get sick about it. I didn't even try to be discreet around my children. They knew he was married but that didn't stop me for a minute. It seemed like I was exhibiting the same behaviors that I had witnessed as a child. Today, I regret exposing my children to these things. Ultimately, his marriage broke up because of our relationship.

When I dated men that didn't use drugs I had to hide my drug use from them. I'm pretty sure they knew something wasn't right. As for the ones that did use, I thought I had hit the jackpot. I never even thought about the damage I was doing to myself. I was at a point in my life that I only wanted men that I could use for money. I guess I had been hurt and disappointed so many times that I didn't care about anyone, not even myself. I loved my children very much but they suffered a lot because of the choices I made. I allowed men to spend the night at my house while my children were home. I thought I was being so smart and yet I was so foolish. Many of my relationships were abusive in one way or another and I continued to get high. I made so many terrible decisions just to get high.

There was a young man who lived across the street from me and he was a big time drug dealer. We had an arrangement that every time he bought drugs he could come to my house and package the drugs for sale. He lived with his mother at the time and she was a minister. In exchange for this he gave me free cocaine. My children were home when he came over and closed himself up in my bedroom. They knew something was going on and you could smell the strong odor of cocaine in the house. The cocaine he gave me was pure and uncut. It was much stronger than what I had been buying off the streets. I thought about getting high more and more. Honestly, getting high was the only thing on my mind.

If I couldn't get cocaine when I wanted it I would drink or smoke weed. I always drank until I was drunk. I never really took just one drink and stopped and this was a pattern in everything I did. When I started smoking cigarettes, I smoked one after another. When I used drugs I always kept going until there was none left and I didn't have the resources to get more. There was a time when I was a regular customer at the pawn shop. I pawned several DVD players. I always planned to go and buy them back when I got paid but eventually I stopped going back for them. It was more important that I got high. As my life continued to spiral out of control I still didn't think I was a drug addict. I thought I was just having fun and I could stop whenever I wanted to.

I wasn't spending enough time with my children and I wasn't consistent with rules or discipline. I was doing my best to take care of my kids but I was so lonely. I wanted to be in a good healthy, loving relationship but I never found it. I was neglecting my responsibilities as a parent. I didn't want to raise my kids alone. I wanted them to have a father and I wanted a husband. I never liked sleeping alone and for many years I didn't sleep at night. I wanted to sleep but instead I lie in bed tossing and turning. My mind wouldn't shut down. I was thinking about any and everything. My past just kept playing over and over in my head. My heart had been broken and I was very sad inside. I was afraid to be a mother all by myself and I didn't think anyone would understand even if I told them. Everyone thought I was strong enough to handle it but I wasn't. I tried asking for help from my family but they weren't willing to help me. Drugs kept me numb and definitely not thinking about life.

I dated many men and it was mostly about drinking, drugs and money. At this point I didn't even respect myself. I was just trying to get what I needed the best way I could. I knew I had children who depended on me and they didn't have anyone else. I knew I had to raise them and I was still high all the time. I may not have been a perfect mom but I was the best I could be and I have always loved my children so much.

I used to close myself in my bedroom getting high while my children were home. When they knocked on the door and wanted something I had to talk to them through the door. I was too high and paranoid to open the door and let them see my face. If they had taken one look at me they would have seen someone very scary that looked nothing like their mom. If it was something they wanted to do outside the house I always said yes. This way they would not disturb me while I continued getting high. I needed help but who could I turn to? My kid's fathers weren't helping and neither was my family. My brother spent time with my children when his kids were around. No one from their father's families had anything to do with my sons and that hurt a lot. They both had great grandmothers who had begun to be a part of their lives but they died early on. I tried to always work and provide for my kids but I had a habit. I wanted to get high every single day.

My sister-in-law introduced me to a man who sold drugs and we hung out at his apartment a lot. Because we were females he allowed us to hang around because we were a good look for him. The conversations always started out very general but would end up sexual in nature. He had a lot of people coming in and out buying drugs while he got high in between sales. Every once in a while he would throw a small amount of cocaine our way. It wasn't enough to get us high but it would cause us to hang around longer hoping he would give us more. I found out that he had been to prison for selling drugs. What if he was raided by the police and I was there? I continued going to his house to buy drugs, hoping he would invite me to stay and give me free drugs. I started going over without my sister- in-law because he wanted to have sex with me. I wasn't interested in having sex with him but I did want to keep getting high. One day I told him I would have sex with him but not at his house. I told him that too many people came in and out and I didn't want anyone in my business. I invited him to come to my house where my children were sleeping. We had been getting high all night and I wanted to keep going but he wanted to have sex. I stalled as long as I could and kept coming up with excuses why we had to wait because I only wanted more drugs. Finally, he became very irritated with me and he was ready for me to pay up. He said no more dope until after sex. I said ok but "let me go to the bathroom first." I went into my children's room and woke up my oldest son and told him to go to the bathroom. I went back into my bedroom and told him he had to leave because my children were awake. He was angry and somehow he knew I had awaked them up but he left peacefully. I was living a life of danger and yet I'm still alive. God had a plan and a purpose for my life and he continued to watch over me in spite of the way I was living. I've heard so many stories of murder and people going missing and this could have easily been me. I thank God for protecting me and keeping me from hurt, harm and danger.

I found a job at a hotel but I was fired for too many call offs. I was high all the time and I couldn't seem to make it to work. I worked midnights and there were times I tried to call off but my boss came and picked me up anyway. I discovered a way to make extra money while working at the hotel. When the guest checked out of a room for the night I went in and cleaned it. This way I was able to rent the room again and keep the money for myself. I used the money to buy drugs. I had regular customers who came every weekend to rent rooms from me. I gave them rates that were lower than what the hotel offered. I called one of my drug dealers to deliver drugs to the hotel. I went in and out of the empty rooms all night long getting high. I even took my dirty laundry from home and washed there and this way I was freeing up more money to spend on drugs. By now my habit was completely out of control but I didn't realize it yet. As long as I had a boyfriend and drugs I thought everything would work out fine.

My next job was working with money. Again, I was stealing money to support my habit. I couldn't take too much because I would get fired and maybe even arrested. One day I stole money from one of my coworkers. She went to the bathroom and when she walked away I quickly went into her cash and stole money from her drawer. After that day I never saw her again because she had gotten fired for what I did. At the time I didn't feel anything but later on I felt horrible for my actions. I was eventually fired as well for no call no show.

My nose burned and would sometimes bleed from snorting so much cocaine. The spirit of addiction is progressive and aggressive and it was gaining territory over my life. I heard about a telephone line where I could meet men. Late at night when I was high and there was nothing on television I called the line. I was looking for men to talk to and meet up with. I recorded a greeting announcing what type of man I was looking for but no one ever responded to that. I was looking for a committed relationship. I wanted to be exclusive and possibly get married one day in the future. When no one responded I recorded a sexual message and the response was overwhelming. Men were looking for women only to have sex with and didn't want any ties. I met several men from this line. I arranged to meet them in public places for the meet and greet. But after that I went to their homes and I even invited some of them to mine. Oh how the Lord has always protected me. I don't know why I continued meeting these men because I was disgusted with most of them. I was hoping to meet a match amongst them but it never happened. Most of them were obnoxious predators searching for sexual gratification. But I still didn't stop calling the line and meeting men.

One day a friend told me she needed to talk to me about something. So I went to her house to find out what she wanted. She told me that her boyfriend and mine had planned to rob a man and steal his drugs. She said we could split the drugs and sell them to make money. Her boyfriend knew the man. They wanted me to go thinking the man wouldn't get suspicious or nervous with a woman in the car. I had never done anything like this before. I guess maybe I didn't really believe it would happen but it did. Before I knew it they both pulled guns on the man and threatened to shoot him if he didn't give them everything he had. What had I gotten myself into? I was terrified and shaking all over. When they told him to get out of the car they began to yell at me to drive away. I was so nervous that I couldn't drive. The man jumped out of the car and started running so I had to get us out of there. I crashed the car and then got stuck in a pile of snow. I was finally able to free the car only to drive into a dead end. I backed out and drove away. I was afraid to go home because I didn't know if we had been followed or not. I didn't know if he had my license plate number and would show up at my house. We went to the liquor store and on the way back we all started using the drugs we had stolen. I was still driving and suddenly the headlights on the oncoming cars got blurry. When we made it back to my friend's house we divided the drugs and my boyfriend and I went home. I never saw our share of the drugs again because my boyfriend stole them from me. I was afraid for my life for a long time after this because I thought this man may recognize my car and come after me. I got rid of the car as soon as I could and I felt a lot safer. I didn't understand what kind of person I had become. Where there were no limits as to what I would do?

    I was using the computer one day and my heart started racing. It was beating so hard and fast I thought it would jump right out of my chest. I was afraid and didn't want to have a heart attack. My first thought was maybe I was having a heart attack from getting high so much. This continued to happen so I went to the doctor to get checked out. The doctor said I was having anxiety attacks and prescribed Xanax for me to take. Of course, being the addict that I was I abused them too. Now, I was snorting cocaine and when I ran out of cocaine and money I took a pill so I would fall asleep. I went into such a deep sleep that I was no longer waking up to send my son to school. He started missing a lot of school. I was mixing alcohol, cocaine and pills and I had no idea how dangerous this was. The devil was trying to kill me but God protected me. I'm so grateful to be alive today and I give God all the glory.

I met a man who lived around the corner from me and he always invited me to his house. He had a bar downstairs and there were always lots of women coming in and out. His basement was like a night club and we drank whatever we wanted and as much as we wanted. He was having sex with so many different women and even young girls that he later told me about. This was disgusting and I was angry when he finally confessed to me that he was preying on teenage girls too. He always wanted to have sex with me but I never did. One day many years after I met him, I wanted to get high so bad and he was my only hope for money so I had sex with him. I thought since I finally had sex with him he would always call me but he never did again. This was a huge blow to the little self-esteem I had left.

    I met a man on my job and I really didn't care for him at first. In fact, we had a huge argument and we couldn't stand to be in the same room together. We found out that we had mutual friends who planned to set us up on a date. Finally, we agreed to go out on a date. I still didn't like him but I went to the hotel with him because I knew he made a lot of money. I was sure this would work to my advantage, so I drank as much as I could before our date. I didn't want to actually remember having sex with him; I just wanted to get it over with. I thought if I had sex with him I would be in a position to get whatever I wanted. My girlfriend and I laughed as we talked because I told her I would have to be drunk to go out with him and that exactly how it happened.

He and I took trips together and it was nice to travel because I had never gone anywhere before. We never did drugs together but he was aware of my drug use and I was aware of his. He decided that on one of our trips he would bring enough cocaine and marijuana to last the entire weekend. I was nervous because I had never done drugs with a man I was dating. I never wanted a boyfriend of mine to know I was using because it was so ugly. When I used drugs I turned into a different person. When we arrived at the hotel I was extremely nervous. I knew he expected us to get high together but I had changed my mind. We sat down and started talking and then he pulled out a bag of cocaine and dumped it into an ashtray. I had never seen so much cocaine at one time and it terrified me. I didn't even want to touch it so I went into the bathroom to get away from it all. I took a shower because we had planned to go to the bar at the hotel to have drinks before bed. But when I got out of the shower he was already so high that he couldn't even talk. He could only make grunting noises and point. I shook my head in disgust and then I joined in and started using too. We never made it to the bar that night because we sat up all night getting high. When morning came we looked and felt awful. We hadn't slept at all and it showed. He suggested that we go out and to get something to eat. We struggled to move around the room in an effort to get dressed and make ourselves look presentable. We found a restaurant nearby and tried to eat but we didn't have much of an appetite. We were there for two days and he had tickets to an outdoor concert for both days. We managed to make it out that evening but it was one of the hardest things I've ever had to do. The events of that day weren't very enjoyable because

I felt so horrible. When we got back to the hotel that evening it was a repeat of the day before only we had more time to get high. It was the worst trip I've ever taken in my life. I saw him change into something very ugly and he saw the same in me. I believe if it had not been for that one night, he and I could have had a lasting relationship.

He didn't like the area I lived in because it was too close to his house where he was living with another woman. He always bought me nice things and took me to nice places. He was good to my children and was a very generous man. One day he told me he wanted me to find another place to live and he would help me pay my bills. He suggested a nicer area in a different city and I was okay with that so I started looking around. I found an apartment in a better community with a better school system. It was definitely more expensive but it would be worth it. He kept his word and paid half of my rent every month. We soon began to have problems in our relationship because he wanted me to commit to seeing only him. I didn't think it was fair to me since he lived with another woman. I never planned to be in a committed relationship with him. I only cared about what he could do for me. Eventually, he started telling me that he was in love with me. Now that I was depending on him to help pay my bills, I felt like my back was against the wall. I insisted that he leave the woman he was living with and he moved in with my children and me. Now instead of going on trips to get high we stayed home and got high. We were both drug addicts and doomed from the start. Prior to meeting him, I was doing smaller amounts of cocaine but now it was on a much larger scale. We often got high for days at a time. Sometimes we went out of town on the weekends just to get high. This way we removed all the interruptions that were around us. We locked ourselves in a hotel room for days using. Sometimes I struggled to breathe as my heart raced because of the amount of drugs I was using. This was very scary but I still didn't stop. I knew that things were out of control but there was nothing I could do to stop it.

We got married and I really convinced myself that our lives would get better but of course it got worse. I thought we would buy a house and live happily ever after but that never happened. I really thought we could stop getting high and build new lives together. I guess my problems were much deeper than I could see or imagine.

He was much better at managing money than I was and he knew how to save too. This was something I had never seemed to be able to do. He worked out a budget for us and I agreed to follow it. I really tried to follow it but I wasn't disciplined at all. He enjoyed getting high and although I was not enjoying it, I couldn't stop using. I was suffering from the spirit of addiction. We got high, paid the bills and had money in the bank. I thought in my twisted mind that things were getting better but they never really did. One day I went to his job and when I drove into the parking lot he was standing there talking to a lady in the car. I drove right past them and didn't say a word to either of them. I knew this was the woman he used to live with. I really didn't know what was going on but I had my suspicions. He didn't know what I was thinking or what I might do so he was afraid to come home that night. He called me on the phone several times trying to see how I would react and when I didn't sound angry he finally came home. I didn't see any reason to argue about it but my feelings toward him had changed. I was angry and insecure and it began to show. Although he managed our finances I still had a debit card. Every time he didn't come straight home I withdrew money from our account. I stayed out getting high until I had spent all the money in the bank. Then I did a horrible thing and cheated on him with another man. I went to visit a friend and we had a drink and dinner. We got in bed and fell asleep and when I woke up it was the next morning. I was afraid to go home because I didn't know what he would do to me. At the time I didn't feel bad about cheating on my husband because I thought he was cheating on me. However, I did feel bad because I had disrespected him by staying out all night. It was only a matter of time before our marriage was over. Because we were both using the marriage never could have lasted. He would get furious when I did drugs with anyone accept him. Even if he knew I was with a family member he still got upset. But as long as we got high together, it was alright with him. One year for Thanksgiving we planned a holiday meal for the family. We took the turkey and ham out of the freezer the night before to thaw out. We planned to have all the trimmings but we started getting high. Of course we stayed up all night and the next day we were too tired to cook anything. We were too paranoid to even leave the bedroom. We sat in the room and let all the meat spoil and had to throw it away. This left us with nothing for our Thanksgiving Day meal and I was upset with myself and with him. At this point I was blaming him for my increased drug use. I convinced myself that if I wasn't with him this wouldn't have happened but that wasn't true. It happened continuously and I was already getting high before I ever met him. After this incident I told him that I couldn't continue to live this way. I had to put my foot down and there would be no more getting high and he agreed. I told him that if it ever happened again he would have to move out. About two weeks later he suggested that we get high and I agreed to do it. I guess I didn't know how to say no because of the addiction. So we got high and after I came down I asked him to move out. I wasn't trying to be mean but I thought if he left I would stop getting high but I didn't.

    I used cocaine with several of my own family members. We used plenty of times together but I guess they didn't suffer from the spirit of addiction like I did. While my drug use got worse it seemed like everyone else remained the same. Eventually, my cousin told my mother and other family members that I was using. No one ever figured out that she only knew because she was using with me. The spirit was isolating me so that it could continue to attack and try to kill me.

Getting high had become everything to me. Everything I did and all my thoughts were related to getting high. I loved my children, my family and myself but I was being controlled by a force of evil and destruction. When I woke up in the mornings I thought about getting high. My appearance, my actions and even the sound of my voice was different. I always felt bad because my kids didn't have what the other kids had but I couldn't help it. I was doing the best I could because I had to have the drugs.

One day my friend and I were going to buy drugs and I was driving. We left the bar together and it was raining outside. I got on the highway and almost immediately, my car was spinning out of control. I could see other cars passing by as we continued to spin until the car landed in a ditch. I called a tow truck and then I called a friend who we had left at the bar. I asked him to come and wait for the tow truck while I used his car to go and buy the drugs. I could have died that day if God hadn't saved me and I still got high. I was hanging out at bars drinking until I could figure out how to get more drugs. I was doing things that were completely out of character for me. Things I would have never done if addiction had not taken over my life. I didn't care what anyone said about me because I had an attitude with everyone close to me. Because they knew I was using drugs I didn't want to be around them. I stayed as far away from them as possible. The only way I was around any one close to me is if they got high too. I never stayed around the same person too long because they would see how bad my drug use was. I had to get high no matter what else was going on.

    I continued to use cocaine and drink excessively. My sister-in-law at the time was a bartender. On days when business was slow she called me to come to the bar to keep her company. I lived nearby and I was glad to do it. Hanging out at the bar gave me the opportunity to meet more people who did drugs. I no longer bought clothes or kept myself up like I used to do. I paid bills and bought minimal food and clothing for my children. The rest of my money went to purchase drugs. My drug use had increased and I was using much more than I had been prior to being married. Somehow I always paid my rent and car payment but I struggled with my other bills. I eventually learned how to work the system. I could get assistance with my gas and lights which freed up money for drugs. I could even get rental assistance because of my income and household size. It may have taken all day sitting in an office filling out paperwork for the assistance, but it was worth it because I could get high when I was finished. I moved into a nicer and more expensive apartment and I still managed to pay the rent there too, at least for a little while anyway. I had relationships one after another and job after job during this time. I was never able to keep a job because of my excessive drug use. I stayed up all night using and when the morning came I was too tired to go to work. Several times I was a no call no show at work. Sometimes I called off so much that I just quit the job because I was too ashamed to go back. For years I didn't realize I was a thief but I was stealing for a very long time before I got caught and went to jail for it.

There was a gas station right outside my apartment complex and the owner gave me a job.

He was married and loved flirting with women so I took full advantage of his lust. I began to steal from him to feed my habit. I gained his trust and he left me alone in the store at which time I started stealing from him every day. I stole food so my kids could eat and I spent more money on drugs. Eventually, I started to steal money too. There were cameras in the store but when I wanted to steal something, I stopped the cameras, took everything I wanted and then turned the cameras back on. I got paid every week in cash and I got high every day. I wasn't eating right or getting enough sleep so I started to look like a junkie. Some nights I sat up all night getting high and I would fall asleep at daylight when I ran out of drugs. I wouldn't show up for work or call off because I had taken a Xanax and was sound asleep. My boss sometimes came to my apartment and rang the doorbell but I never answered it even when I did hear him. While working there I met a man who was a regular customer. Somehow we had a conversation about cocaine. He told me that he had relatives who could get cocaine for him anytime and any amount. I told him that I wanted to sell cocaine for extra money. I asked him if he could get some for me and he said yes. He said he would buy it, package it for me to sell and I could pay him once I sold it. The first time he gave it to me, I did sell some but I used the majority of it myself. He started coming to my job asking for his money and I had to lie to stall for time until I got paid. Finally, pay day came and I gave him the money I owed him and he gave me more drugs to sell. I knew better than to use any of it this time, because I had messed up before. So I didn't use some of it instead I used all of it. The same night he gave it to me I opened the bags one by one until they were all gone. I was so high that I couldn't get up off the floor and I spent the entire night on the floor, on my hands and knees. I was hiding because I thought someone was coming. I never paid this man the money I owed him. One day I went to work and got into an argument with my boss and I pushed him. He called the police but I left before they arrived and I got fired. I was also evicted from my apartment for not paying the rent.

There was a married couple I used to get high with. He got high sometimes but she really liked getting high. She and I started hanging out together and using quite a bit. I didn't have the amount of money she had because she had a very good job. She didn't mind buying drugs for us to use together. She would say "I'll buy, you fly." All I had to do was to go and get the drugs and she paid for them. It was easy to buy them because her brother was the one selling the drugs. If I didn't have enough gas in my car to make the trip, she would tell me to take her car. Even though she and I did lots of drugs together, I guess she didn't have the spirit of addiction. She was still able to get up and function the next day. While she went on with her day I was home sleeping and when night came I was up calling someone else to get high with. One night she and I were parked in the alley behind an apartment building she owned and we were getting high. Our plans were to get high until time for her to go to work and I would go home. But our plans got cut short when a police car pulled up behind us and the officer got out and approached us. The cocaine was on a tray in my hand and she told me to put it underneath the seat. But instead, I poured it out on the floor thinking our chances were better that way. When the officer verified that she did own the property he pulled off. She told me to get the tray so we could finish but I told her it was gone.

    Her mother got sick and I went over several days a week to help care for her. This way she could go to work and not have to worry about her mother. Her younger brother was living there and had recently been released from prison. Her family didn't think he was capable of caring for their mother by himself so I offered to help out. He soon began to show an interest in me. At first I just laughed because he was much younger than me, but I soon gave in to his advances. Although I knew several of her family members I had never met him before. My girlfriend said he was institutionalized. I didn't know what that meant at the time but I later found out. He was a nice looking guy and he loved to flirt with women. He was very disrespectful and everywhere we went he flirted with women and they were flirting right back. Maybe they didn't think we were a couple because of our age difference. He and I fought a lot because he was so disrespectful. All the time we were together he was stealing from me but I was so high that I didn't really pay attention at first. During this relationship God was surely with me and never left me not even for a second. This guy had gone to prison for armed robbery when he was very young. It seemed like every person he knew had gone to prison. He introduced me to his friends and later told me how he met them in prison. I thank God that my children and I are still alive today. If it had not been for God I'm sure it would have turned out differently.

How had I become so sick? It was like a cancer that had metastasized. Getting high was more important than my own self-preservation. I thank God for protecting me and my family and shielding us from danger. One day we were drinking and getting high and his married cousin came over with another lady and they went downstairs. I knew his wife and one day after that incident, I had been drinking and drugging and I unintentionally told her what had happened. I never planned to reveal his secret but because I was so full of alcohol and drugs it just slipped out. She was furious when I told her what I had witnessed her husband doing. She got in her truck and went driving around looking for him. When she found him she starting shooting at him while she was driving down the street. I thank God nobody got hurt that day. When he found out that I was the one who told his wife he vowed to kill me. My boyfriend told me that this man had killed several people and I shouldn't have betrayed him. Months after this happened I got a phone call that this man, who vowed to kill me, had shot himself. I prayed and asked God to comfort his family because I knew his mother, wife and five children. One day my boyfriend and I had an argument in front of his friends and he hit me and ran away. I chased him but I couldn't catch him, however, I was determined to get even with him. He called me on the phone soon after the incident and wanted me to pick him up so he could spend the night with me. He acted as if nothing had happened but I hadn't forgotten about what he had done. I went and got him but he had no idea of the danger he would face that night. I had endured years of physical abuse at the hands of many men and I wouldn't be beaten again. When we got back to my apartment I acted as if everything was fine. It was time to go to bed and I let him get undressed but I kept my clothes on. I walked out of the bedroom and went and got a hammer. When I started to open the door he must have seen the hammer in my hand. He tried to slam the door in my face but the struggle was on. I was trying to force the door open and he was trying to keep it shut. Unfortunately, I was able to get the door open just enough to swing the hammer and hit him in the head. Blood splattered everywhere in the living room. It covered my shirt, the couch and the walls. My youngest son was there and he took the hammer from me at which time my boyfriend came out of the bedroom. He grabbed my car keys off the table and I grabbed the nearest object to try and stop him from leaving with my car. I threw the iron at him but it missed and he ran down the stairs and out the door. He drove off in my car and I was furious. I picked up the hammer and left the apartment walking. I walked down the street with the hammer in my hand and blood on my clothes. I was out of my mind and definitely not thinking at all. I knew that when I found him in my car he would regret it. He lived quite a distance away from my place. It was about a two hour walk to his house but I didn't care how long it took me to get there. I was very angry and I wasn't thinking rationally. I was determined to find him that night. While I was walking I kept calling his house but he never answered. I kept walking because even if he wasn't there he would show up eventually and I would be there waiting. I decided maybe I'd better check the hospital first because he was bleeding very badly. Two men in a pickup truck stopped and asked if I needed a ride and I said yes. I wasn't even thinking because of the rage inside of me. At the time I had no fear at all inside of me. I thank God they dropped me off at the hospital unharmed. I saw my car parked in the emergency room parking lot. I went in and walked up to the desk and asked if someone would go to the back and ask him for my car keys so I could leave. I didn't even ask how he was doing and didn't even consider the fact that I could be arrested on the spot. One of the nurses went to the back and asked him for my car keys but he refused to give them to me. I had no choice but to wait for him to be treated and released. Finally, I saw him walking out with his head bandaged. His head had required several staples to close the wound. A police officer was with him and they were walking straight toward me. The officer asked me if I had hit him with a hammer and I said yes. I explained to the officer that he had hit me a couple of days prior and ran away. As the officer listened to my side of the story he looked down at the ground and shook his head. He just turned and walked away without saying a word. I asked for the keys to my car but he still wouldn't give them to me. He knew that if he gave them to me I would get in and drive off leaving him there. He got in the car first and then let me in. That night we went back to my apartment together. The next day I felt horrible about what I had done and I knew this relationship had to end. I started crying out to God asking him to remove this man from my life. My whole life could have been over in an instant. I thank God that I didn't kill him with that hammer. I'm glad my son was there to stop me but at the same time I was sorry he had witnessed the incident. I would never want to live the rest of my life in prison and with murder on my conscience. I don't understand why I didn't just walk away from him.

I came into some money and we decided to sell drugs. I wanted to sell cocaine and he wanted to sell crack. We drove to his cousin's house to buy drugs. I gave him the money to make the purchase and he went in the house but never came out. He had left out the back door while I waited for him in front of the house. He disappeared into the night so I went back to his house to see if he would show up there but he didn't. I called the police and made a report that he had stolen some money from me. Of course I didn't tell them that the money was to buy drugs because they might have arrested me too. A warrant was issued for his arrest and he was picked up and taken to jail. I received a check in the mail for the full amount he had taken from me. Finally, this relationship was over and I was indeed very glad.

I had to move again. This time I moved to a very large apartment complex. This was not like any place I had ever lived before. My ex-husband came over to see our son and he said "oh you finally moved to the ghetto." I was angry about the comment but it was true. There were people walking around and just hanging out all day and night. After living there for a short time I started hanging out too. I was alone and wanted to meet someone and make friends. This place was infested with drugs and drugs addicts. My ex-husband had always told me never to try crack cocaine and I never did until now. I was still using cocaine but everybody I met was smoking crack. I tried hanging out with them and asking if they could get cocaine for me. They told me the dealers in the area only sold crack. Maybe they only told me this hoping I would buy crack so they could have some too. One day I asked one of the ladies if I could try smoking crack with her and she said no. She really didn't want me to try it. I thought she was being greedy and wanted it all for herself. But I can remember the look on her face when she said no. I realize now that she was trying to save me from the evil spirit but I would listen. I needed to get high and if crack was the only thing around I was willing to try it. I also tried heroin on two different occasions and I thank God I didn't continue with that. I was so messed up that I was willing to try anything that would get me high. I was getting high with a couple one night and we ran out of crack and it was too late to buy any more. They had heroin and the man offered me some and I said yes. His girlfriend was against it and upset with him for even offering it to me. But he said a little wouldn't hurt so I snorted it. I was so high on crack that I don't know how it made me feel.

I met a lady who was friends with a friend and she had prescription medications for pain and mental illness. One day we ran out of crack and she offered me some pills and I took them. I didn't even know what they were or how they would affect me. If it hadn't been for the mercy of God I would have been dead. I was reckless and foolish and there seemed to be nothing I wouldn't try. Suddenly I had no control over my life. I didn't know who I was or what I was doing but I kept right on doing it. When I wanted to use I had to call one of these so called friends I had met and have them buy the drugs for me. Of course, I didn't know what I was doing so they had to show me how to use this drug. Slowly I began to meet drug dealer's right there living in the same complex as I did. Two of them lived right next door to me so I didn't even have to leave my apartment to buy drugs. I was getting high all night and sleeping all day. When I woke up I was thinking about getting high again. The spirit of addiction had totally consumed me. It was all I could think about day and night. Nothing else existed from the moment I first smoked crack cocaine. All of my waking hours were spent thinking of ways to use. I remember asking the Lord to please help me to understand what was going on inside of me. When I wasn't high sometimes I just walked through my apartment screaming and crying out asking God to help me. I didn't want to do what I was doing but I couldn't stop. I didn't know how to stop. I didn't even know who I was anymore. I looked different, acted different and indeed I was different.

    I was driving home from a club one night and my car stopped in the middle of the road. I was drunk with an open bottle of liquor on my back seat and I had a bag of dope in my pocket. The police cars drove up behind me and the officers got out and approached as I sat in a drunken stupor. The officer asked me what had I run into and I told him I hadn't hit anything. According to him I had hit something. I think somewhere in the fog I remember some front end damage to my car. I really don't know what happened. A police officer drove me home and they never even gave me a breathalyzer or searched me. I didn't even get a ticket and I know this had to be the favor of God. The next morning I woke up fully clothed and as I sat up slowly in bed my mind was cloudy. I sat up and looked out the window because for a moment I thought I was dreaming. But when I saw my car wasn't there I knew it had really happened. Suddenly as bits and pieces of the previous night started to come back to me I was terrified. I didn't know what I had hit and I could have been in some very serious trouble. I could have killed someone and I didn't even remember what happened. I knew I didn't want to live this way. I didn't know if the police would knock on my door and take me to jail in the next second.

This was when I decided that I would leave my car at the tow yard and let it be repossessed. I had been making payments for more than four years. The car would have been paid off in six months but this would be best until I got my life together. I had to get off drugs and alcohol. I never saw that car again and I was sure I had done the right thing. A story began to circulate that I had pawned my car to a drug dealer. I was exhausted from living this lifestyle and I wanted to change. I wanted to live a normal life and didn't have the strength or desire to defend myself against any accusations about me. I felt good about my decision and I figured this was a small sacrifice if it meant me getting my life together.

I dated a married man for several months and every time we got together we got high. He was able to find cocaine and we snorted it together all the time. When we got high I couldn't go to sleep so I always asked him to stay a little while longer. He only came around when he wanted to get high. He knew the dealers and I spent all the money even though he made more money than I did. One day he called me and wanted to get high but I told him that I needed to pay my bills. I needed a ride so I asked him if he would come and take me and he said yes. He picked me up and he kept talking about getting high but I insisted on paying my bills. He called a drug dealer and told him to meet us because he wanted to buy drugs. I thought he was going to buy them but when the dealer pulled up beside us he asked me for the money. I told him that I wasn't giving him any money. The drug dealer got very angry and pulled out a gun and threatened me telling me not to play games with him. I could have lost my life that day too but God had a plan for my life. Even though I was going through awful things he was there protecting me the whole time. I was still in the car with him and he cursed me out the whole time. This is when I found out that he smoked crack because he starting smoking while he was driving. I began to cry and I was so afraid. It was midday and we were on a very busy street. He finally took me back home and dropped me off but eventually I started smoking crack with him. He soon began having trouble in his marriage. He called me one day and said he couldn't see me for a while. He had to go straight home after work until things calmed down. That was fine with me and I just kept getting high. By now he had introduced me to several of his friends who smoked crack. They started visiting me and we got high without him. Crack was a lot easier to find than cocaine and everybody else was smoking crack. When no one came around the women I had met in the complex were always available to buy crack for me. I gave them the money and they called a dealer to bring us the drugs. I really didn't have any idea what I was doing so I always got very little of what I bought but I kept buying it anyway. No matter how little I got or how bad it was I kept buying it. I lived alone so my apartment was the spot to come to when they wanted to smoke. I guess the street law was if someone smoked crack in your house they had to share whatever they had with you. It was very irritating because I only got a small fraction of what they had but I did it anyway. I was so desperate to get whatever crumb I could to get high. As I continued to smoke I began to get bold and I would approach their dealers when I saw them in public. I asked for their phone numbers so I could call them for myself. I wouldn't have to share my drugs with anyone but this turned out not to be such a good idea because I fell deeper into addiction.

Men were always propositioning me and being very disrespectful. I hated it but I guess I looked and carried myself like what I was. Besides that I was disrespecting myself. I wasn't getting along very well with the women I had met because they started sleeping with my male friends. I felt betrayed so I stopped hanging around them. There seemed to be so much confusion everywhere I went. Being alone wasn't good either because I only had more time to do more drugs. I needed to come up with more ways to get more money to do more drugs. I've never known anyone personally who's overdosed. However, I do know that I consumed so many drugs that only God could have kept me alive. There were times that I got high all alone for days. I locked myself in the apartment and closed the blinds then it was just me and the crack. I wouldn't answer my phone if it rang and I wouldn't answer the door if someone knocked. I looked different and sounded different so I didn't want anyone to see me. I wasn't bathing, brushing my teeth or eating. The only thing I could find the strength to do was get high. I started using early in the morning just as soon as the dealers got up and I used all day. The only reason I stopped was because I ran out of money or the dealers ran out of dope. Sometimes they just went to sleep and stopped answering their phones. At that point I would lay there looking at the clock and hoping the time would go by faster so daylight would come and I could buy more drugs. I was crying out to God but I kept on using. I was asking God to make me stop but I guess he didn't hear me. Once I had been getting high for days and I clearly remember crying and screaming asking God for help. Using drugs was the basis of every decision I made. When I went shopping it was so I could get done with it to get back home to get high. When I did have a job I always went to work high. When I got off work my focus was on getting more drugs.

My sister came over one day and said that God had assigned her to me. I didn't know exactly what that meant but I was willing to listen. She asked if there was anything I needed from her and I told her that I wanted to go to church but I didn't have transportation. She told me she would get back to me with the names of some churches that had vans and could pick me up. Eventually, I went to her church because she was married to a pastor at the time. I went to church and continued using. Some days I was picked up by one of the church members and other days I rode the city bus to church. I wanted very much to come out of this lifestyle so I kept going to church. One day I rode the bus to buy drugs and went to church with the drugs in my pocket. I felt lower than dirt and I was terrified to bring drugs into God's house. I didn't know if He would strike me dead for this but He didn't and I'm so grateful. A lady at the church gave me a bible and I started to read it. I remember reading a scripture that talked about when an evil spirit leaves it would return with seven spirits more evil than the first. I began to scream and cry out to God. I continued to scream for a very long time and I fell to my knees because I knew that I wouldn't be able to handle this. How could I possibly handle seven more evil spirits? One day I had an urge to use but I tried to pray my way through it instead. I was hoping that if I prayed to God and asked him to help me I wouldn't use but I still used that day. There was another time that I didn't want to use so I sat on the couch and put the bible next to the telephone. I wanted to call for drugs and I wanted to call God. I wanted Him to stop me from using so I picked up the bible and I held on to it tight. I asked God to stop me from calling the drug dealer but I called anyway and I kept on calling. I continued to meet drug dealers in the area that I lived in so I always had someone to call.

A friend of mine from high school who had moved away came to visit one day. When we were in high school he always had a crush on me but I never felt the same way about him. He invited me to come to visit him in Birmingham. He offered to buy me a round trip airline ticket so I said yes and was very excited to get away. While I was there we were drunk every day. I even blacked out a couple of times from all the drinking and partying. I wanted some drugs because alcohol and drugs went together but I didn't mention it to him because he didn't use drugs. When the trip was over and I came back home he started calling me saying he wanted me to move to Birmingham with him. I was all for it because it seemed like a chance for me to get away and start all over leaving this nightmare behind me. I was very excited but no one was excited for me. The people at the church were saying it was not of God for me to go and live with a man I wasn't married to. My family was concerned about how he would treat me once I was there. I wasn't concerned about that because I knew I could take care of myself once I got there. So I looked at the move as a stepping stone for me to begin a new life. Even if he and I didn't work out, I could get my own place and I would be fine. I thought that just maybe this was God's way of getting me out of the environment I was in. I discovered that I didn't know God at all because this was not his will. Fornication is a sin so this couldn't have been God. I began to pray and ask God to help me and lead me in the right direction. I started packing my bags and throwing things away that I didn't want to take with me. I had arranged for my son to take over my apartment because it was more suitable for him. I really didn't know if everyone else was right or if I was right so I just kept preparing to move. Then one day I went to sleep drunk on my living room couch and I was dreaming about moving when suddenly I heard a loud voice say "No." I immediately opened my eyes and looked around but no one was there except me. I had never heard God speak but I thought this had to be Him. I was uncertain about what had just happened so I prayed, "God I think I just heard you tell me not to move but I don't know for sure. "I need to be sure that I'm doing the right thing so I'm asking you to make it crystal clear." I kept packing until I got a phone call from my friend in Birmingham saying that he had changed his mind. He no longer wanted me to move there with him. I knew that this was God making it crystal clear just like I had asked. I wasn't sad and I didn't cry about it. Maybe I was a little disappointed but I was thankful that God didn't allow me to make that mistake. I kept going to church and I kept getting high.

One day I got on the bus and the driver looked very distressed. I asked him if he was okay because I saw pain on his face. He told me that he was going through something and didn't want to talk about it. I tried to encourage him by telling him things would get better. When the bus stopped he began to tell me that he was a married man who had been cheating on his wife for a long time. He said he wanted to tell her of his infidelities. My advice to him was not to tell her but to stop cheating and be faithful to her. My intentions were pure and good but I eventually dated him too. He told me stories about his crack addiction but insisted he had been clean for some ten years plus. I believed him even though he and I were drinking every night. He said he would rather kill himself than to ever use drugs again. He also said that he would never be around anyone who used drugs and especially not a woman. I only used when he wasn't around so he wouldn't find out about the addiction I was battling. I wanted him to keep coming around because he didn't mind spending money. I believe the spirit of manipulation started to rise up in me at this time.

I can remember the exact moment our relationship began. We had only been friends and together we talked about things that were going on in our lives. He told me to demand respect from men and not to accept anything less. He told me the type of man he was and that I should look for a man who was willing to take care of me. I was hungry one day and asked him to buy me something to eat. When we walked out of my apartment I smelled something awful. I couldn't identify the smell but I had never smelled anything like it before. I didn't say anything to him right away. We walked outside to get into his van and when he opened the door for me I smelled it again. I asked him if he smelled anything and he said no. When he opened his door I smelled it again. I knew I wasn't losing my mind and I knew that the smell wasn't coming from me. I didn't think it was coming from him but I didn't understand it at all. If I had to describe the smell I would say it smelled like something rotting. It was like the smell of death and I believe it was an evil spirit. If I had been in the word of God and in right relationship with Him I might have known what I smelled. I might have taken heed of this warning and been spared the excruciating pain of this relationship. This was a sign to get away from this man. But I was with him for several years and the relationship was very toxic. He bought my food and told me to keep the change which was about $20.00 and that's a lot for a crack head. He started giving me money all the time and soon after that he started asking me for sex.

One day he was visiting me and we were drinking with mutual friends. Another guy had given me some crack and I was waiting for my date to leave so I could smoke it. Finally, he left and I didn't walk him to the door because I was ready to start smoking. He let himself out while I was in my bedroom sitting on my bed too drunk to move. As soon as I heard the door close I started smoking. Before I knew it he was standing right in front of me. He said that he had been suspicious so he hid in the closet by the front door. He caught me red handed and began to curse me out, calling me every name in the book. He turned and stormed out of my apartment and I locked the door behind him this time. He called me in a couple of days and told me he was clean and would have no further dealings with me. I understood and really didn't care because it was more important for me to get high than to date him. Later that same day he called again but this time he had a proposition for me. He said that if I agreed to stay in the house at night and promise to only smoke crack when he was there he would buy it for me. If I would agree to these terms he would buy all the drugs I wanted. This way I wouldn't have to call anyone to bring it to me and

I could keep my own money. This sounded like a great deal to me so I agreed. Because he had smoked crack before he would certainly understand my struggles and be able to help me stay in control. Of course this was not realistic because crack heads can never get enough. I was spending every dime he gave me and my own money too. He came over one day and bought everything I needed to smoke with. We sat at the table and he taught me how to smoke crack. It didn't take long before he and I were smoking together. At first, I blamed myself that he was using again but later I realized it wasn't my fault. Several people including my drug counselors told me that if he were truly clean he would have never given me the drugs. He blamed me that he was using and his family also blamed me for his so called relapse. I guess they never thought about the fact that he used for years before he met me.

Several of his immediate family members were drug users as well. His family was just as dysfunctional as mine if not more. I wanted out of this nightmare.

I stopped going to church and was high all the time. I cried many days because I didn't know what else to do. I didn't have the strength to do anything other than smoke. One day I was in the shower crying and when I got out I called a lady I knew and asked her to pray for me. I was surprised and thankful that she didn't even ask me what was wrong. She just began to pray and I still got high after that. I never saw anybody or talked to anybody. I was too paranoid to face people whether they knew me or not. It was even difficult to face the dealers when they delivered the drugs so I looked at the floor while making the transaction. I couldn't stop getting high even when I wanted to. There were times that I had been getting high for days and I was so tired but I still wanted more drugs. I didn't want people to know how much I craved the drug so I went from person to person getting high. I can only imagine what the dealers thought about me because they knew the truth. I always spent all the money I had and called them constantly until I was completely broke.

One night I had been getting high all night and I finally fell asleep in my son's bed. I was home alone and when I woke up something was speaking to me and I think it was God. He told me to get up and get the telephone book from the closet and look up addiction. I called a number for a treatment center and they said I could come to the center that same day. I was very excited and suddenly I had hope again, until they said it was in Florida and then my heart sank. I was a crack head living in Indiana and we don't ever have money because we spend it all on drugs. I told them that I didn't have any money to purchase a plane ticket and they said they would call me back. When they called back they told me they would buy the ticket and I could pay them back at a later date. I asked if I could come the following day and they said yes. I called my dad and asked him to take me to the airport and he was more than happy to do it. I packed my bags that included my bible and a book my sister had given to me. The book explained how God has a purpose for all of our lives.

The next day my parents dropped me off at the airport. I remember feeling relieved and anxious at the same time. I was eager to get the help that they were offering me. When I arrived in Florida someone picked me up at the airport and drove me to the center. I had to be checked in and when I was assigned my room, I went straight to sleep. I knew God had sent me there because my spirit was so peaceful and I wasn't afraid at all. In fact, I was excited to get help with my drug addiction.

Everyone I met there seemed to be having a difficult time. People were asking me to pray for them and I had never prayed aloud or in front of anyone before. But I couldn't tell them no, so I did the best I could. I didn't have to detox or take any medication for withdrawals. I met with counselors, therapists and medical staff while I was there. We had group sessions and also had local pastors visiting on Sundays to talk with us. One of the counselors told me that talking in group would help me to heal. I told her I didn't want to share all the sordid details of my life with everyone. But she explained that this was the time and the place to tell all. I was surrounded by others in addiction just like I was. They were from all over the world and I would never see them again. I decided to take her advice because I no longer wanted to be sick and I didn't want to die. I started talking in group and I told everything. I told them that I was a liar, thief, cheater and prostitute. I talked about my past in detail as everyone stared on. I could see them whispering but I didn't care. It felt good to release all the turmoil that was overflowing inside me. A weight was being lifted off my shoulders so I kept talking every chance I got. Eventually, we started attending meetings in the community and I did the same thing there. They called it sharing in these meetings and I had no problem sharing my story.

I was quickly progressing in the program. People were coming up to me saying they wanted to do the same thing. I encouraged them to share their stories and experiences. I told them how good it felt to let it all go. It wasn't long before I was moved into an apartment which was part of the program. There were four beds in each apartment but they only put one person in the apartment with me. We were picked up daily and taken to the treatment center to attend group and counselling. We also ate our meals there too. My roommate and I didn't get along very well and I don't know why. I tried to get along with her but it wasn't working out. During one of the group sessions, I explained the problems we were having and asked if we could have alternative housing arrangements. She said she would speak to the director about our situation. My roommate felt the same way I did. They ultimately decided to keep us together and said that we had to figure out how to get along. I didn't understand at all because they could have easily separated us. But for some reason they chose to try to force us to get along. One night I called my mom crying and she suggested maybe I should come home. I didn't want to come home. I wanted to finish the program so I would be done with drugs forever.

Things never got any better between my roommate and I. We eventually got into a huge fight inside the apartment. She was taken to the hospital and I was taken back to the facility and isolated from the others. Ultimately, I was told that I had to return home. I was being kicked out of the treatment program and I couldn't believe it. I was so upset that this happened and I didn't know what I was going to do. I couldn't go back to the same lifestyle I had left behind. They said they would give me a referral to a treatment center near my home but I declined the offer. I had only been there about three weeks and it was a 90 day program. I was angry with the director for refusing to move us and I was angry at myself. I was afraid to go back home. I didn't want to start using drugs again but a feeling was starting to rise up inside me. I was embarrassed that I had gotten kicked out of the treatment program. I was very much afraid that I would use again. There was a very real voice inside my head telling me "since you got kicked out of the program, you may as well use."

A part of me thought I could make it because I had done so well in the program. I would take everything I learned while I was there and apply it to my life. I had to find someone to sponsor me and I needed to attend AA/NA meetings. For a short time I really thought everything would be alright. But as I sat in the back seat of the car on the way to the airport, fear was raging inside of me. Someone was talking in my ear. I couldn't see them but I heard them loud and clear. The voice was telling me to get high when I got home. It was the devil and he wouldn't stop telling me to use. I didn't want to use but the voice was winning. He wouldn't stop talking to me even thought I didn't want to hear it. He didn't shut up all the way home and by the time my plane landed, I was ready to get high. Finally, I arrived home and it was pretty late at night. My parents picked me up from the airport and I went to their house for the night. I was relieved because I knew if I went back to my apartment I would be overcome with my past. I was terrified at the thought of going back to that place. I had to change people, places and things in order to stay clean. The next day my parents suggested that I live with them for a while. That was sweet music to my ears and I was so grateful. I quickly moved everything out of the apartment. I put my things in storage and moved in with my parents.

I found an AA meeting right away that was nearby. I went to one meeting but I didn't like it very much. When the meeting was over I walked to the bus stop and a man followed me. We had just left the meeting and he was drunk. In the meetings they advise you not to get in a relationship for at least one year after you get clean. This man clearly wasn't following this suggestion.

It wasn't long before I found a meeting that I enjoyed going to. Every time I went to a meeting and shared I cried and I couldn't seem to control it. I was tired of crying and I seemed to be the only one sobbing all the time. It was so embarrassing so I didn't share as much as I wanted to. I started thinking about using again so I called the treatment center. I left a message asking a counselor to call me back but I never received a call. How could they treat people as though they cared but once we left they forgot all about us? It would have been nice if there was a crisis line to call but I didn't have that option. The majority of the employees at the treatment center had suffered in addiction at one point and time. Didn't they realize how afraid I was? I was in trouble and likely to use again if I didn't find help. I was all alone in my struggle to stay clean.

I started going to meeting a couple times a week. There was a NA meeting in the basement of a church. I sat and listened for a while and slowly I began to talk to the people in the room. I needed a sponsor and one of the men offered to sponsor me until I found a female sponsor. There was an apartment building next door to the church where they sold drugs. This was very uncomfortable and tempting for me but the fear of getting caught stopped me from approaching them. My dad helped me get a job and I was so excited. I was also very optimistic because I was clean and going to meetings. I had a sponsor and a job so things were looking up for me. I was living safely with my parents and saving money. I was riding the bus to the meetings and to work but I was getting tired of it. My parents were both retired and I thought they could have helped me since I was trying to do better. I thought they could have given me a ride sometimes but they never did and I didn't ask.

I was riding the bus every day and eventually I ran into the same man who was buying drugs for me. I started dating him again. I worked at a pharmacy that sold liquor. I was excited because I hadn't had a job in a long time. I worked at the liquor counter and addicts are taught in the program to stop drinking, drugging and using mind altering substances. My sponsor told me that I shouldn't work at the liquor store. But I told him that I was fine and I wasn't drinking. I really believed I could stay clean and sober. After all wasn't it God who had sent me to the treatment center? Hadn't God given me the job too? One day I decided to get a wine cooler and I thought there was no harm in it. It didn't take long and I was drinking hard liquor and soon after that I was using again. I was still living at my parents' house so I bought a bag of dope every now and then. Of course, it didn't stay that way for very long. Once my parents saw the same man coming around my mother told me I had to move out. She saw me going back to my old ways and she was not going to tolerate it. I was angry because she was right but I wasn't ready to move out yet. I had planned to live with my parents for a year but it had only been six months. I found a place right away and I moved out. I had saved up enough money to pay first month's rent and security deposit. I bought brand new bedroom furniture and paid cash for it. I still had money in the bank which I planned to use toward the purchase of a car. I completely turned to the married man because I felt as if he was all I had. He was attentive to my every need and he spent a lot of time with me every day. He was good at pretending he cared about me but he was only manipulating me. He always did nice things for me. He gave me rides to and from work and he even let me use his car sometimes. Some days he sent his friend to pick me up so that I wouldn't have to ride the bus. He seemed to be the only one who cared about me. He always gave me plenty of money. He got my hair done every two weeks along with pedicures and manicures. These were things that I never had before. He spent time with me every day after he got off work. He always made sure that I had everything I needed in the house. I had never had a man to fulfill my every need. He always told me that he loved me and I believed him. I thought he really loved me or I guess I wanted to believe he did. Maybe I felt this way because I had no one else who seemed to care about me at the time. Maybe I didn't even know what love meant. Everyone in my family was upset with me because I was using again. They seemed to be more concerned with themselves than about me and I was the one who needed help. He and I continued in this relationship and I soon began to ask God to separate us. Once again I couldn't seem to just walk away. I really tried to but I kept going back to him. If I left him for good I wouldn't know what to do with all my time. I didn't want to be alone all day every day. Who would pretend to care about me then? I thought it was better to have someone to pretend to care than to have nothing at all. I didn't want to live in sin and I didn't want to cause him to sin either. But I couldn't seem to just walk away.

My head was spinning so fast and I was exhausted. I would have preferred that he was faithful to his wife but I couldn't stop seeing him. God knows how tired I really was. I was beginning to see that he didn't love me at all. When I saw him he encouraged me to keep doing the right things. I confessed to him that I was drinking again and he was okay with that. He said that he didn't believe drinking would lead me back to drugs but it already had. I hid it from him as long as I could. I kept saving money until I was ready to start looking for a car and he helped me do that too. We looked at a lot of cars but I didn't have enough money for the cars I really liked so I kept looking. I finally found a good running car that was affordable and I bought it. I was so proud of myself for all that I had accomplished. Now that I had a car I could go buy drugs whenever I wanted to. Soon after this I stopped going to meetings. I was spending time with this man and when he went home I left out right behind him going to get high. I didn't know he was parking around the corner watching and waiting for me to leave. He had been following me and I never realized it. He had known all along what I was doing.

I lived around the corner from my parents and they owned the house next door. Their tenants moved out and my mom called and asked me if I would move into the house. She said it would be good for me to live next door because they were getting older. I was fine where I was but I agreed to move into the house and it was a huge mistake. My decision to move caused an even bigger division between my family and me. After I agreed to move in I found out I would be paying the same rent as everyone else. I had assumed since I was their daughter I would get a discount on my rent. I guess I should have asked that question before I gave up my apartment. Since there was no mortgage on the house I wasn't expecting to pay the same as total strangers had paid them. I regretted moving into the house and I stopped speaking to my mother. I was getting high more and now that I lived right next door, my parents could see a lot more. There was traffic in and out with my boyfriend and drug dealers. I was running back and forth all day and night buying drugs. My lights were on all night and the blinds were closed all day. I left home to go to work and when I got off I bought drugs to take home with me. Sometimes I had the dealers bring the drugs to my job so I could go straight home. In the beginning my parents occasionally knocked on my door but I never answered. I was either too high or sleeping off a high. I didn't want them to see me that way so I hid and eventually they stopped knocking. I was spending money as fast as I could make it so I needed to figure out how to get more money. A friend of mine introduced me to his friend who was a drug dealer. He was very nice to me in the beginning. He even bought me flowers once and he always gave me drugs when he came over. He smoked weed and drank but he didn't smoke crack. In the beginning it all seemed so innocent but then he started to hint around that he wanted to have sex with me. I was all for it thinking how nice this arrangement would be but he changed after the first time we had sex. A part of me actually thought he liked me. But he started talking to me like I was nothing but a crack head. He stopped giving me crack and demanded that I have sex with him in exchange and I did. I never liked doing it but I had to because I craved the drug. I hated the way he treated me and the way he talked to me. But I continued to allow myself to be disrespected and degraded for drugs. He no longer came over to talk and he only wanted to see me when he wanted to have sex. During this same time there was a man I met on my job. I think in the beginning he really liked me but I wasn't interested in him other than for money. After I spent all my own money getting high I tried calling one of these men to make more drug money. I was smoking up my pay check along with the bill money. My mother was angry with me because my rent was late a lot. She was putting late notices in my mailbox that she had my sister to type up. I couldn't seem to stop smoking long enough to do anything else. I had a coworker that needed a place to live and I came up with the bright idea to rent my basement to him. He had two jobs and we rarely saw each other. There was a problem because his rent was always late. I was getting upset with him because I counted on him paying on time so I could get high. He had a girlfriend who used to come over sometimes. But then she stopped going home and was there all the time and he still had not paid rent. I heard that they were going to move into an apartment together. I felt like he was trying to use me while he saved money to move out so I kicked him out.

I met a lady on my job that needed help doing her income taxes. I tried to explain to her how easy it was for her to do it herself. She still wanted me to do them for her and she was willing to pay me. The first year I filed her return and when she received her check in the mail she paid me $100. The following year she came to my job and told me that she wanted me to do them again but she didn't have the money to file. I told her she could file them and have the money deposited into her bank account and they would deduct the fees. But she didn't have a bank account so I filed her taxes and had the refund sent to my account. I was only trying to help her while helping myself at the same time. The sooner I filed her return the quicker she would receive her check and pay me so I could get high. Her state refund came first and I took the money to her house. She told me she would pay me after she received her federal refund. I was disappointed because I thought I was getting high that day but I said okay. When the federal refund deposited into my account I decided to borrow $100. I could get high and then replace the money when I got paid. Then I would give it all to her at the same time. I withdrew the money and I kept withdrawing money and getting high. I knew I was in trouble because I couldn't stop using. I got high all day and night for two days straight. I knew it would take me longer to pay her back than I had originally planned. I knew

I would need more time to get all the money together so I lied to her. I told her that the money had not come yet. This plan went all wrong because I was fired from my job and I had no way to pay her back. I was already in so much trouble so I kept using until all the money was gone. I didn't work there anymore so I wouldn't have to face her. She didn't know where I lived but she did have my phone number and she started to call constantly. I changed my number so she couldn't contact me. One day I walked outside my house to talk with a friend and there she was walking toward me. I looked at her and at the same time she looked right at me. She approached me and started screaming about her money. I took her inside and told her that I would pay her soon.

Over the next month I sent her a money order for $100. My intention was to repay her every dime that I had stolen from her. That proved to be impossible because I kept buying drugs. One day I was sleeping and I was awakened by a knock at the door. I had been up all night using so I peeped through the blinds and saw a police car sitting outside. I composed myself enough to open the door. When the officer saw the door open, he came to the porch and asked my name. I told him who I was but I wasn't sure why he was there. He told me that I needed to come with him. I asked him what would happen if I didn't go and he said he would arrest me. So I knew I had to go no matter what happened next. I put on some clothes and got in the back of the squad car. When we arrived at the station he put me in a room and walked out. I sat there quietly wondering what would happen next. Finally, someone came into the room and started questioning me about the income tax money. I told him that I had not paid her because something unexpected happened. I told him that I planned to repay the money and had never planned to steal it. I tried to convince him that I was telling the truth so I told him that I had given her the state check. I also told him that I gave her a $100 money order. He walked out of the room and when he came back he told me that I was free to go home. I later found out that she was also at the station in another room. I was relieved when I was taken back home. I planned to pay her back as fast as I could. Unfortunately, I let another month go by and I didn't send her any more money.

I started receiving mail from lawyers offering to represent me. At first I didn't think anything about it but the letters were flooding in. This prompted me to call one of the attorneys and to my surprise there was a warrant for my arrest. My bond was $1,000 cash and I would have to be booked into the jail. I had never been to jail before so I decided to save enough money to bond myself and then I could turn myself in. But instead I smoked every dime I got my hands on. My parents told me to get out of their house because I hadn't paid rent in almost two months. My son had moved in with me so I told him to find a place and I would help him with his bills until I left town. I had enough of this place and the way I was living. He found an apartment and I moved out of my parent's house and in with him. I thought it would be hard for the police to find me since I had a new address. But one day I went to buy some crack and on the way back home I was pulled over by two police officers. They already knew about the warrant so I was taken into custody. They let me call my son to come and get my car so they didn't have to tow it and I was grateful for their kindness. They never found the drugs in my pocket because I was able to get rid of it before they searched me. At least I no longer had to live with the threat of going to jail in the back of my mind because now I was there.

I was put into a holding cell where there were several women already in custody. I found a place to sit as I waited to see what would happen next. I didn't want to talk to anybody and I tried to keep to myself. I didn't know if I could take being locked up in this place. After several hours I was taken out to be finger printed and allowed to make a phone call. I called my mother and told her where I was. I was taken back to the cell where I remained for the next two days. There was a toilet in the middle of the cell that we all had to use. I held out as long as I could before I used that toilet.

Finally, I was taken from the holding cell to the jail and it was even worse. They assigned me to a cell and I went inside and looked around in a daze. I was finally able to take a shower which felt wonderful because it had been days since I'd had one. They gave me a pair of paper panties to put on. I just wanted to break down and cry but I fought back the tears. I was afraid to let anyone see me cry. I lay down on the bed and stared up at the ceiling as I fought back the tears. Even though I didn't want to kill myself, I was so tired of living. I couldn't imagine ever being able to make it out of jail in my right mind. I knew there was no way I could stay locked up in a cage like an animal. I just couldn't wrap my mind around what I had gotten myself into. I didn't think I was strong enough to last inside these walls. Suddenly I saw a picture of Jesus inside the light fixture. I don't know if it was actually, physically there but I know what I saw. At that moment I felt stronger and I knew I would be able to hold on until I got out. I had told my son not to worry about getting me out of jail. I knew I was wrong for what I had done and I needed to face the consequences for my actions. I had told him to take my check and pay my part of the bills but I changed my mind. I wanted him to get me out as quickly as he could. I was locked up for five days and on that last night my son came and bonded me out after midnight.

Thank God I was free and this had taught me a lesson. I would never go back to jail because I would live right and never use drugs again. However, on my way home I asked my son to stop at a friend's house so I could get some sleeping pills. I told him that I wanted to get a good night's sleep but I lied. I went inside the house and bought some crack. I hadn't been out of jail thirty minutes and I was already using again. I never thought this would happen but I felt like I couldn't go home without it. I was so messed up and I knew only God could help me. I was hoping he wouldn't let me die this way.

I was given a court date and a public defender. My lawyer told me how angry the prosecutor was about what I had done. He said they were not willing to make a deal with me. It looked like I would be serving time in jail for theft. I asked my lawyer if he realized this was my first offense and he said yes. He told me that he didn't understand why the prosecutor was being so hard on me. While I waited for my court date I continued reading the bible and getting high. I read a scripture that said don't think about what I should say and God would give me the words to speak at the right time. I kept repeating this to myself so that I would not get nervous or afraid. Finally, it was time for me to stand up in front of the judge and talk. I told the truth and trusted that God would do what he said he would do. I had faith that God would work everything out and he did. I never confessed to being on drugs. I simply told the judge that I didn't plan to steal her money. I said that things happened that were out of my control. He didn't want to believe this was my first offense but it was the truth. I was relieved when he decided to give me probation for one year. This was actually a felony but somehow I was assigned to misdemeanor probation.

When I met my probation officer I was embarrassed because I was the oldest one there. The worst part was that I was still getting high. My probation officer told me that I had to follow the conditions of my probation or I could be incarcerated for up to one year. I was not allowed to drink alcohol or use drugs and I would have to submit to random testing. I couldn't even go inside a bar and could not leave the county for any reason. I also had to report to my probation officer once a month and repay the money I had stolen. There were also probation fees that I had to pay. I knew I couldn't go back to jail so I had to stay clean, but I couldn't. I came up with a plan where I could get high for the whole month and stop one week before my probation appointment. The problem was that I couldn't stop one week or even one day before. I just kept using and one day my probation officer handed me a drug test kit. My heart sank because I knew I wouldn't pass the test. There was no reason for me to waste the test so I confessed to her that I had used. I told her I was smoking marijuana instead of the truth about my crack addiction. She decided to give me a break and not violate me. She warned me not to let it happen again but I couldn't break free from the drugs.

I was assigned a new probation officer and I saw him several times. He never mentioned drug testing me so I got real comfortable getting high. My probation was almost over. I thought I was home free but then he asked me to take a drug test. All I could do was tell him that I couldn't pass the test and he gave me a break too. At this point I asked him if I could transfer my probation to Minnesota. I wanted to leave the area to get clean. My niece and nephews lived there and had been asking me to move there for years. They agreed to the transfer but first I had to pay all the fees that were required for the transfer. I would also have to live with relatives there. My niece didn't have room for me to live with her so I asked my nephew if I could live with him and his family and he said yes. They completed the necessary paperwork and filed it. I paid the fees and was preparing to go when my probation officer informed me that they changed their minds for some unknown reason. They refunded my money and I used it to smoke crack. I had been looking forward to leaving, getting clean and having a new beginning. But now that I wouldn't be going I was so distraught. I would have to wait until my probation was over.

When I finished probation I wanted to leave but for some reason I was still hanging around. My family in Minnesota called me asking why I wasn't there. I don't believe it was time for me to leave at that moment. My dad's health was declining and I really didn't want to go. Furthermore, it was scary because I would be leaving everything I had ever known. I found another job and I don't even know how I was working because I was high all the time. I was living with my parents again so I stayed out all night getting high and came home at daybreak. I wasn't getting much sleep before going to work which made it very difficult to function. We did a lot of sitting in the car all night smoking crack and going to cheap motels.

One day I went to work after being up all night using. My boyfriend dropped me off at work but he called off that day. He called me before it was time for me to get off and he was crying. He said that he had been getting high all day and he and his wife were fighting. He said that he couldn't go back home that day. He wanted to stay in a hotel but neither of us had any money. My pay day was the following day so I asked my boss if she could pay me in advance and she did. When I got off he was outside sleeping in his truck so I got into the driver's seat. I stopped at my house and grabbed some clothes for work the next day. After that I went and bought some crack so I could smoke once we got to the hotel. I was hoping he would go to sleep and I could have it all to myself but we got high together. When all the drugs were gone I tried to get some sleep so I could go to work the next day. He started talking about killing himself and asked me not to leave him. I didn't know if he really would have or not but I called off anyway.

When I woke up the next day I was exhausted from the lifestyle. I knew I should not have called off and I knew I had let my boss down after she tried to help me. I was ashamed for what I had done and I knew it would be difficult for me to face her again. I started pacing the floor and talking out loud to myself. I asked myself why I was still in Indiana. I should have been gone to Minnesota a long time ago. I tried to come up with a reason why I had stayed so long but I couldn't. I knew I should leave because there was no reason not to. I was procrastinating and delaying my health and healing. I felt like I should leave that very day but he was telling me that I couldn't just pick up and move away. I asked him why not? I got a message from my boss saying she was suspending me for two days. We left the hotel and he dropped me off at home. My mother and sister were at church and my dad was in bed watching television. I walked into his bedroom and said good morning and I could see that he was irritated with me. He said "I thought you were moving to Minnesota?" At that moment I knew it was time for me to go. Suddenly I had no fear, no hesitation and no worries. I got on the phone with my relatives in Minnesota and asked if I was still welcome there and they said yes. I told them I would be there in two days and I would phone later with my arrival time. I went downstairs and started packing and throwing things out. I rode the bus to go and buy my ticket. I was finally leaving and I needed to find someone to take me to the bus station. I called my boyfriend first and he said he couldn't do it. I asked my sister for a ride and she said she couldn't do it either. She suggested I leave on a different day but there was no going back now. I refused to get frustrated or discouraged. I went back to my sister and asked her to drop me off early and I would spend the night at the bus station. The terminal was big and scary because I was there all alone but I had to go. I knew I had to stay awake and alert because anybody could walk in at any time. But God is so good because he didn't leave me there for long before he sent a police officer to watch over me. A squad car pulled up and parked outside and stayed there all night. The officer never even got out of the car. When morning came my bus pulled up and I boarded.

When I arrived in Minnesota I was excited to see my family. I was thrilled to be in a different environment where no one knew me or my past.

A place where I didn't know any drug dealers and didn't have to hold my head down in shame everywhere I went. I sat around talking with my family getting caught up and settling in. I had not let go of the married man I had been dating and getting high with. I was talking to him the entire time and immediately we planned a trip for me to go back and visit.

I lived with my brother's ex-wife and her husband. They were very nice to me and did everything to make me feel comfortable. Immediately I started taking care of business. I went and signed up for low income housing and I started applying for jobs. I was living in the house with a pastor and they had their own church. I was glad to go to church on Wednesdays and Sundays. I was trying very hard to get closer to God. I wanted to know who God was and I wanted a relationship with him. My family in

Minnesota was very close knit and always came together in fellowship. More importantly, they all knew and loved the Lord so this was great for me. I was going to church, taking notes and asking questions but I didn't understand much of what was being said. After church was over everyone stood around talking and I started to feel left out. They had been together for so long and shared many memories and good times and I wasn't a part of that. I didn't know how to join in with their conversations. I wasn't used to having a family that got together and actually talked and laughed instead of fighting. I quickly started to isolate myself from them. I felt like I didn't fit in anywhere. I started to wonder why I was so messed up that I couldn't even fit in here. Something had to be wrong with me but I didn't know what it was. I tried to change so I would fit in but it wasn't working and I didn't know what else to do.

My boyfriend wired me some money for a bus ticket. While I was in Minnesota, I got clean but I couldn't wait to go back to Indiana to use again. As soon as I bought my bus ticket I started getting anxious to use again. When I arrived, he picked me up from the bus station and took me to a hotel. I told him I wanted to get high. He tried to talk me out of it but I insisted so he bought crack for me. We got high the rest of the day and spent the night together. The next morning he went to go to work and I just stayed at the hotel all day until he got off. I didn't even go and see my parents but I did see my sons. I was only in town for a couple of days and when the time came to go back, I wanted to stay with him but he said no. When I returned to Minnesota I continued to go to church. We visited different churches where

God would use people to talk to me. People that I didn't know would come up to me and tell me that God said to "trust him." I thought I was already doing that but apparently I wasn't.

I cried a lot a night and I thought no one else knew it until one day a pastor told me that God sees my tears. He told me to trust God. It touched my heart to know that God was watching me cry at night. I knew God was real and I had to know more about him. I began to pray to God but I didn't think I knew how to pray the right way. The enemy had convinced me that I wasn't doing it right so God wouldn't listen to me. This was a lie from the pit of hell. I tried to sound like other people when I prayed but it was too hard. I thought to myself that maybe it would be best if I didn't pray until I knew what I was doing. I realize now that all God wanted was for me to talk to him but at the time I didn't understand that. All I had to do was go to God with a sincere heart and talk to him and he would listen. I hadn't realized yet how much He truly loves me. I believe God was starting to change me.

I had started talking to my dad on the phone and he was excited that he was getting stronger. I was planning to travel back to Indiana for another visit. My dad wanted me to see all that he could do on his own and I was looking forward to it. But he was admitted into the hospital before I made it back to see him. The day I arrived I didn't go to the hospital because I started getting high. But the second day I went to the hospital and he barely woke up. He told me that he was in a lot of pain so I told him to rest and I would come back later to check on him. I left and it wasn't long before I got a phone call that he was getting worse so I went back to the hospital. The doctors told us that we needed to say goodbye and dad died that day. Mom and I left the hospital together and had a disagreement before we were half way home. I told my mother that I wanted us to be closer. I let her know that she had hurt me over the years but she didn't want to hear it. So I left it alone and it was quiet in the car for the rest of the ride. I stayed with my son while I was in town because this way I could spend more time with my boyfriend. Mom asked my sister to speak at dad's funeral and to write the obituary. I was angry and hurt because she didn't ask me to do anything. I'm not sure that I wanted to, but it would have been nice to be asked. I didn't think I should have been excluded from being involved with planning our dad's funeral.

One day mom asked me to clean the kitchen and my aunt was visiting. They sat at the dining room table talking. Mom was cleaning dad's jewelry when I heard her say she would give it to my nephews and my brother. I walked into the dining room and looked at the jewelry and asked if I could have a gold chain and she said, no. Mom said she was giving it to my nephew. Then I asked her if I could have anything that belonged to my dad and again she said no. She told me that I could have something of hers when "she was dead." I exploded and began to cry uncontrollably. I told her that he was my father and I felt like I should have something of his but she still said no. I stopped washing dishes and went to get my things and I walked out of the house. It was raining outside and I was a long way from my son's house where I was staying. I called my boyfriend who was working at the time. I rode the bus to his job and he gave me a ride to my son's house. I had no intention of talking to my mother again because this was just too much for me. I had made up my mind not to attend my dad's funeral because I was drained from all the confusion. I was very upset and I missed my dad so much. I felt as if I had to protect myself from my mother because she said such hurtful things all the time. I didn't call her and she didn't call me. I didn't hear from my brother or my sister. This too was very hurtful because no one seemed to care about me. My oldest niece did call and talk to me every day. When she finally arrived in town she never left my side. I had one girlfriend who stayed in contact with me and helped me to get through this difficult time. I told her all that had happened with my mom and that I was not going to the funeral. She said that I had to go to the funeral even if she had to force me. She offered to go with me so that I wouldn't have to be alone. I'm grateful for everything she did for me during this time. She picked me up and took me and bought me something decent to wear to the services for my dad. My son, niece and I rode to the funeral home together. When my sister saw me sitting there she walked up to me and hit me in the head. I was furious and raised my hand to hit her but she caught my hand. She hadn't even called me and all she could think to do was hit me? I didn't go anywhere near my family because I was upset with them. I kept my distance from them while I was there. A couple of relatives spoke to me but most of them didn't. At one point I saw my mother heading in my direction and I went the other way. God only knows what she wanted to say but I couldn't take a chance on her hurting me again. When the wake was over my niece and son wanted to go to my mother's house. I didn't want to go but I didn't want to be the cause them not going. I rode along and sat in the car until they were ready to leave. There were people outside talking so it wasn't awkward for me to be there. My cousin came up to me and said I should go in the house. How could she know what I should do? She didn't know what was going on because our family doesn't communicate with each other. Sometimes they won't even speak to one another in public. She had never come to visit my mother or father or even called for that matter.

Waiting for the day of the funeral was difficult for me. I cried all the time and I got high and drank a lot too. I had a friend drive me to my aunt's house and I sat and cried as I talked to her about how I felt. I told her everything that had been going on. She suggested that I contact my uncle because he had been looking for me. We drove to his house and he was glad to see me and I was equally glad to see him. We talked about my dad and I told him the things my mother had said to me. I was expecting him to have some gentle, comforting words but I was shocked at what he had to say. He told me to grow up and get over it. He basically said that I had spent too much of my life trying to have a close relationship with my mother. He said it would never happen and I should love her and move on with my life. I didn't know it then but soon after I realized this was what I needed to hear. I had to move on and I could no longer be stuck trying to please my mother. No matter what I did it would never be good enough for her so I had to live my life. She was satisfied with the way things were between us and she said it all the time. She's always said she didn't like my ways and I should change. I don't know who she wanted me to change into but it was time for me to move on. I had to accept this because I didn't have the power to change the way she felt. I would still need time for it all to settle in my mind and I knew it may take a while. It was still very hurtful but at least I knew what had to happen.

When the day of the funeral came my son, niece and I rode to the church together. We were already there when the funeral car arrived. I heard them announce that it was time for the family to go outside and line up to walk in the church. I didn't bother going out, instead I stood inside and waited until they walked past me and I followed behind. I sat in the church behind them and I felt safe where I was. I just wanted this day to be over. After the funeral I rode to the cemetery with my aunt and uncle. I got out of the car and walked to the grave site. My mother, sister and brother were already seated and there was a chair for me. My brother asked me to sit beside him and I did. As I walked away I grabbed a flower off the casket and put it in my bible and kept it there for the next two years. I never got a picture or anything to remember my dad so I put his obituary in my bible. It's still there today and I'll always keep it right there.

I stayed in Indiana longer than I had originally planned. I never talked to my immediate family again during that time. One day I was riding the bus talking with a lady that I had previously met. She wanted to know why I was back in Indiana. I told her about my dad and all that had happened between my mother and me. She told me that God told her to let me know that in a few months my mother would call. She said when we talked not to mention anything from the past. I stayed for about a month before I returned home to Minnesota. I traveled by bus again but this time the ride seemed longer than usual. My family in Minnesota thought I wasn't coming back. It was more difficult now because not only had I moved away but now I had lost my dad too. I knew I couldn't continue to travel back and forth. I had to settle down and adjust to my new life.

I started looking for a place of my own and I searched even more for a job. I found a job but it would be a challenge to get there. Since I didn't have a car I had to depend on public transportation and family to get to work. I was dropped off and picked up during my week of training. Fortunately, it wasn't too far from home. When it was time for me to start the job, it was quite a distance away. It was at least a thirty minute drive and I would have to ride the bus and the train. My nephew's wife picked me up and dropped me off at the train station every morning. It was very early and still dark outside when she dropped me off. I waited for the train which was all new to me. When it finally came I got on hoping I would reach my destination safely. I listened as each stop was announced and when it was time for me to get off I was nervous. I got off and walked down the stairs and out of the station looking for the bus I would have to ride. I saw one parked on the street so I walked over and asked the driver for help. I told her the address where I needed to go and she told me that my bus would be coming soon. She said it would pull up on the other side of the street. It wasn't long before the bus did pull up and stop. I gave the driver the address of my job and he told me to get on. He said he would let me know when I arrived at my stop. When he stopped for me to get off he pointed me in the right direction. He told me I was about two blocks away from the address I was looking for. I thanked him and started walking. It was still dark outside so I looked closely at the addresses on the houses. It didn't seem as though I was headed in the right direction but I kept walking. I walked for a while checking for the address but I still didn't see it. I had a feeling something was wrong but then I thought, maybe I just don't know the area. I tried to use my cell phone for directions but it wouldn't work. It had always worked before so I didn't have a clue what the problem could be. I walked for probably an hour until the street cut off because there was a school in front of me. I didn't want to get lost so I decided I'd better turn around and go back in the same direction I had come from. Meanwhile, I tried to call my job thinking they could give me directions but no one answered the phone. Again, I tried my phone for directions but it didn't do any good. The sun was coming up and I was so tired from walking. I started talking to God asking him why this was happening to me. How could I be lost in this strange place all alone? I was afraid that I would be lost for a while and I didn't want to lose my job for being late on the first day. I wanted to cry but I didn't. My legs were hurting and I was so discouraged but I still wanted to show up for work. Just when I was ready to give up and go back home, I found it. I explained to my coworker what happened and she took me outside and showed me that the train station was within walking distance from the job.

Every day was a journey getting to work. I got up at 3:00 am and I didn't have to start work until 7:00. I arrived thirty minutes early daily because of the train schedule. After work I rode the train to the mall where I caught a bus and still had to walk twenty minutes to get home. When I finally did make it home it was about 6:00 pm and time to get in bed to rest up for the next day. I didn't communicate with my family in Indiana and not too much with my family in Minnesota. I started isolating from everyone. I started to cry a lot more than usual and I didn't know why. I curled up in bed at night and cried like a baby. There was no one to tell and no one I could talk to. I seemed to be the only one who had no relationship with anyone. This troubled me especially when I saw how close everyone else was.

I started stopping at the liquor store on my way home from work so I could drink myself to sleep. I was so lonely and it hurt so badly. I felt like I was in a world all alone. My life was dark and empty and I only existed in it because I had to. I think when my boyfriend stopped calling that was the final straw because no one was left in my life. I felt like I was dead on the inside. There was nothing there but darkness, emptiness and so much sadness. The crying spells were increasing and happening everywhere I went. I cried at the grocery store and even at the doctor's office. One day I cried at the doctor's office and I tried to explain to her how I felt but I really didn't even understand it myself. She offered to prescribe medication for depression for me to take but I refused. I had been praying asking God to save me and I wanted to trust and depend on Him. After all that's what everyone kept tell me, "trust God." I wanted to trust and depend only on Him. I had been going to church and listening to what was being taught. I was also praying and spending time talking to God and He was talking back to me. I knew it had to be Him but I didn't fully understand. I only knew that I wanted to get to know Him better. She gave me a phone number for a psychologist but I never saw him either. Instead I went to church and when it was altar call, I ran to the altar and dropped to my knees. I began to cry out to God begging Him to help me. At that moment, there was no one in the room except God and me. I felt as if my head would explode with everything that was going on inside of me. I needed the Lord to help me right then because I couldn't go on any longer. I grabbed my head with both hands as I cried out to the Lord for help. My brain felt like it was filled to overflowing. There were so many thoughts inside my head that it spinning around and around. I couldn't open my eyes and I couldn't stop crying out to God. I asked God to take away whatever was trying to destroy me. It seemed as if something was trying to take control of my mind and my thoughts. This couldn't happen to me. At some point I got up and went back to my seat where I continued to sob quietly. I didn't notice anything different right away but I soon realized that the crying had stopped. I believe with all my heart that God had done this for me.

My doctor suggested that I exercise to clear my head and relax and I thought it was a great idea. I joined a health club and I started walking. I didn't know the area so I had to find a route that was comfortable for me. I walked every day and it was very relaxing. There were always lots of people out running and walking their dogs. I thought I would lose weight and even though I didn't I kept walking anyway. Sometimes my great nieces and nephews wanted to walk with me but they were really too small. I took them sometimes because I enjoyed the company. At times I felt closer to the little ones than I did the adults. I thought since I didn't know anyone in the area, my niece and nephews would embrace me but they didn't. I didn't see them very often and they didn't call me. I was really hurt by it all but I tried not to let it show. I tried to focus on starting over with a life that didn't include drugs. I was hoping when I found my own place I might not feel so rejected. But the apartments were so expensive I couldn't afford one of my own. My niece suggested I explore the option of having a roommate. I considered it but soon abandoned the idea. Since I felt excluded from family events and planning I started doing everything by myself. I went to the movies and out to eat alone. I walked to the strip mall to get out of the house and keep myself busy.

As soon as I started walking I began to have issues with my knees. Every time I tried to take one step forward I was knocked back ten. Would anything ever work out for me? I found a doctor who specialized in knee pain and I made an appointment. He took some x-rays of my knees and hips. He gave me a cortisone injection and a knee brace to wear whenever I had to stand for long periods of time. The injection relieved some of the pain and I wore the brace when I worked.

Six months went by and it was time for another injection. But this time it didn't last as long as the first one did, so the doctor had to look at another course of treatment. He recommended a hip specialist who determined that I needed a hip revision. I had been in contact with my mother and sister for a couple of months by now. I called them and told them of my upcoming surgery. My mother and sister made plans to come to Minnesota to be with me when I had surgery. The surgery was scheduled and I took medical leave on my job. My family arrived the night before my surgery and I spent the night at the hotel with them. We got up early the next morning and headed to the hospital. When I woke up from the anesthesia my nephews, their wives and children were all in my room. I was heavily sedated and unable to stay awake but I was glad they were all there. The next day my mom and sister had to go back home and they stopped by to see me before they left. I stayed in the hospital for three days and then I went to a rehabilitation center to recover. After spending five days in rehab I had hoped to hear from someone in my family but I never did. Finally, my youngest nephew called and my niece and her children stopped by to visit for a second.

I was in a place where I didn't know anyone except my family and they didn't even check on me. My pastor came to see me on more than one occasion. I had run into an old school mate from back home and he came to visit me too. I was so depressed and hurt that I didn't want to leave rehab but I had to go. I didn't have anyone to pick me up so I called a cab to take me home. I had to stop and get a toilet seat lifter and shower chair on the way and the driver was kind enough to make the stop. When I got home no one was there so the driver helped me carry everything inside. Soon my sister-in-law came downstairs to apologize for not calling or coming to visit. I didn't want to talk to her because there was no excuse for not even calling me. I didn't respond to anything she said. She told me that they would be moving out of the house and into an apartment then she walked away. My niece came right behind her and I let her know how upset I was. I cried as I told her that I felt so mistreated by her and her brothers. She cried too and I know she was hurting but I was tired and just wanted to get some rest. I told her we would talk later and she walked out of the room.

The next few weeks were challenging because I had doctor and therapy appointments scheduled. I couldn't drive for six weeks because of the pain medication I was taking. I was too angry and rebellious to ask for a ride so I arranged for medical transport to pick me up. I was discouraged because I had believed God for a place of my own which I still didn't have. I knew I had to go back to Indiana if I didn't have a place to live soon. They were moving into a two bedroom apartment. She did offer me the spare room but I no longer wanted to impose on them. Beside I wouldn't have any privacy and neither would they. I didn't know what would happen to me. But one day my great niece came downstairs and told me that she would miss me when I left. My first thought was that God was telling me I would be moving but I needed to be sure. I talked to my sister and she confirmed it was time for me to move back to Indiana. She told me to be patient until she could get some days off work to come and get me. Because I had recently had surgery she brought a friend of hers to drive my car back. The last thing I wanted to do was go back to Indiana and fall into my same patterns. I was hesitant because I would have to move into my mother's house. Although we were speaking I knew it wouldn't be easy for us to live together. The last think I wanted to do was go there. When they started packing I did too. I asked my nephew and his wife if I could stay with them for a few weeks while I waited for my sister to come. When she arrived we loaded up both cars and drove back and I moved into my mother's house.

The moment I had completely recovered from surgery I started looking for a job. I found the same company I had worked for in Minnesota. I had to reapply for the job and they hired me right away. A background check and license check had to be completed before I could begin. I was home waiting to receive my work assignment when I got a letter rescinding the employment offer. I was disappointed but I kept looking for a job. I submitted several applications online and even went on some interviews. I was hired on two different occasions but those offers were rescinded as well. I registered with more than one temporary agency but they didn't call either. I was sitting around the house everyday doing nothing with no one to talk to. I was very lonely and getting depressed. I started smoking crack again because I couldn't take it anymore. I tried many different things to occupy my time but nothing seemed to work. I tried calling family members who didn't want to be bothered. They wouldn't even return my calls. I tried spending time with my grandson but that was difficult too. I don't know why I thought smoking crack would take away the pain because it didn't. I knew if one of the agencies called me for a job they would drug test me but I kept using.

One day an agency called and wanted me to start a job immediately. They asked if I could come in to take a drug test that same day but I knew I couldn't pass it. I told them I was out of town and wouldn't be back until the following week. I was disappointed in myself and I began to shut down completely. I was so depressed that I could barely move. I cried a lot and stayed in my room all the time. I kept going to church and I kept praying when I wasn't high. I didn't want to live this way and I didn't know what to do.

I was asking God to save me and I desperately needed His help. Somehow, I stopped getting high long enough that when the agency called again I was ready. I was so happy to finally have a job again. My birthday was coming up and I invited my sons, grandson and sister to dinner and I was paying. This was something I had never done in my life and I was so proud of myself. I enjoyed our time together and afterwards I took my grandson and bought him some toys. Everyone went home and I was alone again. It was still early and I should have gone home but I didn't. I called a friend and told him I was coming over. I stopped on the way and bought crack for the two of us. I stayed there smoking until it was too late to buy anymore then I went home. I had to work the next day and although I wanted to call off I didn't. I felt and looked horrible and I couldn't wait to get off so I could go home and get in bed. I went on a smoking binge for the next couple of weeks.

When I lived in Minnesota I deleted all the phone numbers of the people who had anything to do with drugs. But as soon as I made the decision to use, their phone numbers popped right into my head. I hadn't used these numbers in two years but instantly I remembered them. Things got bad quickly and I was using every day I could. I was spending all my money getting high and I was sneaking around to do it. I parked in our driveway and lay down across the front seat of my car smoking crack. I didn't want my mother or any of the neighbors to see me. I was afraid that I would burn my hair and I probably did but I kept smoking anyway. If I knew my mother wasn't going outside I could smoke in the garage. I had to be careful because if she came out to get in her car she would smell it. At the time my mother owned the house next door and we used the garage for storage. I used to pretend that I had to go inside the garage to look for something but I was going to smoke. Sometimes after I was done smoking I was too paranoid to come out of the garage so I stayed inside. One night I was in the house but I wanted to use so I made up an excuse to leave out to get high. I was running in and out of the house until about 10:00 pm. I knew I had to stop around that time so I wouldn't arouse suspicion in my mother. Sometimes I was so desperate to use that I thought about climbing out of my bedroom window in the middle of the night. I never did only because the house sits high up and I might have gotten hurt or awakened my mother.

I was awake all night because of the drugs in my system. I fell asleep at day break for only a couple of hours and then I started smoking again. I couldn't get as high as I did before because I wasn't working. I didn't have anyone buying drugs for me and I wasn't in contact with the people from my past. I was disappointed and upset with myself because I was right back where I had started. I couldn't stop and I felt pitiful and sickened by the things I was doing. Although no one knew the details of how I was living I couldn't hide from myself. I was so ashamed that it was eating me alive. There couldn't be anyone more sickening than I was. I felt hopeless and I was so tired of living this way. I thought no matter how hard I tried or what I did things would never get better. I was going backwards and I wondered what it would take for me to be free from this demon. I heard that you have to hit rock bottom before things can start to change. How could I possible go any lower than I already had? How could I talk to anyone about what was happening to me?

God gave me the strength to go back to church. Even though I was still getting high I felt like there was still hope. I tried to go to church every Sunday but sometimes after being up all night getting high I couldn't make it. I started going on Wednesday nights when I could. I really wanted my life to change and God was the way to do it. When I wasn't in church I was thinking about getting high all the time. I kept going and sometimes I invited other people to come with me. I wasn't really learning that much but I kept trying because I wanted to know all about God. My youngest son's father (the one that beat me) invited me to his church and I went there too. The people at my church were somewhat unfriendly. They laughed and talked amongst themselves but only a few of them even bothered to say hello. I never stayed and mingled after church was over, I left right away.

One day I called the church and asked to talk with the pastor because I needed someone to pray for me. I was told that the pastor was unavailable and that someone would be in contact with me soon, but no one ever called. I was still using and I wanted it to stop. I was crying out for help but there didn't seem to be anyone willing to help me. I was so desperate to talk to someone who could help save me. I remembered I met a pastor at my aunt's wedding. I looked for his phone number and I called him. I thank God for reminding me of this pastor because he was available. He told me to come to the church so we could talk. I went immediately and I started talking and crying. I can still remember the look on his face as he sat and listened to everything I had to say. Of course I didn't confess that I was on drugs but God had probably had already told him that. When I was finished talking, he prayed for me and I left.

I continued to go to church and use drugs; I thought it would never stop. All I wanted at this point was God in my life. I didn't want the drugs anymore. I didn't want or need a boyfriend either. I didn't even care what my family thought or said about me. I needed God to save my life. I thought if I joined a ministry in the church then I would stay busy and drug fee. But in order to join a ministry I had to take the new member's classes that were eight weeks long. It took me even longer because when I was high I didn't go to church but I finally finished. Then I found out that I had to take additional classes that were introductions to each ministry.

One Sunday the pastor announced that he wanted to start a ministry for drug addicts. I was interested in this because there were others in the church who had been delivered from addiction. We had a meeting with pastor and planned to start the ministry. But then it was postponed because it was anniversary time at the church. I was discouraged because of the delay but there was nothing I could do. During our pastor's anniversary we had several guest speakers. They took up a lot of offerings and I gave as much as I could. I even gave what I didn't have because they promised that I would get it back but I didn't. I gave from the money I had set aside to pay my car insurance. He said that God would give it back and multiply it but that didn't happen and my insurance lapsed. I always wanted to be a tither and a giver but this confused me. After this happened I was afraid to give anymore. I just didn't know what to do. We gave so much that the pastor said "God told me not to take any more money from the people." We constantly gave honor to our pastor and his wife. Everyone stood up and clapped for the both of them. They stood up and clapped all night long for the pastor and I didn't think it was right. On the last night of the anniversary the pastor was not there but they still stood up and clapped for him. That's when I walked out of that church and I never went back again.

One day I talked to my sister about how I wanted to have faith. She told me that faith comes by hearing and hearing by the word of God.

I decided I would go to church as often as I could. I watched church on television and listened to it in my car. Because I was still getting high I knew I had to find a church nearby so I wouldn't have an excuse not to go. I found a small church that was within walking distance from my house. They had bible study on Friday nights and I started going. Sometimes I went to this church on Sundays too. I also found a church that had bible study on Tuesday nights and it was even closer to my house so I went there too. I also went to church with my sister on Thursday nights. One Sunday I went to church very broken and I asked one of the ladies to pray for me. I know it was God who led me to ask her because I didn't even know her. She said "I'll get the pastor," but I told her I needed her to pray for me. She called one of the other ladies over and the two of them prayed with me. I found out these ladies had a prayer group that got together once a week. They invited me to come and even though I had no idea what was involved I went anyway. I was afraid not to go because I needed every connection to God I could get. I went to prayer and it was at someone's house. I met them there and I sat on the couch as they prayed. I didn't know what to do so I just listened, watched and cried. I kept coming back every week and eventually I started praying with them. I'm not positive what was happening as I began to pray but I believed I was being loosed.

One day I talked with one of the ladies and told her that I needed to find a church because I wasn't really satisfied where I was. She invited me to visit her church and I asked where it was. When she told me the name of it I knew I couldn't go there. I wanted to visit this church before but I heard they would require me to show my W2's to them. I knew I wasn't making any money and I didn't want to be embarrassed. I thought you had to be rich to go to this church. I used to pass by the church and see all the nice cars in the parking lot. I wanted to be like them but I thought I'd better save myself from being rejected. She told me it wasn't that way at all and I really wanted to go. I didn't want to go alone so I invited a friend to go with me and she agreed to come. Sunday morning about an hour before service my friend told me that she wasn't coming. I was so desperate for God that I had to go so I went alone. I sat through the service and the following Sunday I went back and joined the church. At this church they were teaching about living a life of faith. The pastors were teaching and I was learning. It wasn't long after that when I realized that I wasn't craving drugs anymore. Not only that but I wasn't craving cigarettes or men anymore. I wasn't even using foul language. I knew this had to be God and I'm so grateful. I had been crying and trying to quit on my own for so long and nothing seemed to work. God is able to do exceeding and abundantly above all I could ever ask or think. He brought me out of the darkness and the hell I had been living for so many years. This whole cycle started when I was very young but that didn't matter to God because he loves me so much. I give God all the glory for delivering me from the hands of the enemy.

I have to keep going until I get to the place where God wants me to be. I believe he was trying to get me to this church for a very long time but because of the rumor started by the enemy, I was in fear. The enemy had me convinced that I wasn't good enough. When everyone else had given up on me God never did.

I had to keep my mind occupied so I wouldn't relapse. I prayed and studied the word. I went to church and tried to live according to the will of God. I tried to make changes in the things I used to do. I worked on having a better attitude and treating people better than I had in the past. I asked God to help me and to guide me. I could see some changes taking place in my life but I had a long way to go. I wanted to be content with who I was and where I was in life. I was finally on the right path seeking God instead of everyone else. I struggled and wavered between trusting in people and trusting in God. I knew that I should lean and depend on God alone but I didn't know how. All my life I had put my trust in man and it ended in disappointment every time. It wasn't easy trying to change my way of thinking. I finally realized that I needed to ask God to renew my mind. I will never stop seeking Him. The bible says that our faith cannot waiver and we must remain faithful to God. So many times God used people to tell me to have faith. I prayed and asked God to increase my faith. I told God that I didn't have the wisdom to do it myself. Then I prayed and asked Him to give me wisdom. I know there is nothing I can do without God. I kept praying and asking Him to help me and I knew He would. The bible says keep asking, keep knocking and keep seeking and I won't stop until the door is opened. I was exhausted from all the ups and downs.

I trust in the Lord with all my heart because if it wasn't for Him I would be dead. God says that He will comfort me in all my troubles and I understand that He was always with me. I have to make things right with every person that I have wronged if and when the opportunity presents itself. Lord, if I've said or done anything to hurt anyone I repent today. Lord, I pray that you will teach me how to always treat others in a loving and kind way. Teach me how to help others and not hurt them. Make my words kind, gentle and loving when speaking to others. I strive to be more understanding of others no matter what they say or do. Lord, show me how to be kind to my enemies. Father, I ask you in Jesus name to teach me to be patient and kind. Teach me how to fight evil with good. Forgive me Lord when I fall short of the goodness of your glory. I have to remind myself that God loves me and he weeps with me. You said that you will turn my tears to joy and I thank you Father. I can rejoice because I know God has prepared a place where I will weep no more. Lord, please help me to remember that I am not alone and that the Holy Spirit is the Comforter. I want to live my life in a way that when I die people will remember the good I've done and not the bad. I will work diligently to please God so that my good far outweighs the bad. Thank you Lord because you have forgiven me of my sins. Thank you for teaching me how to forgive others. I will always depend on God for all that I need because this world is not my source.

I am an ambassador for Christ and I will always tell others the Good News of Jesus Christ. In everything I do and say I want others to see the good in me. When people look at me, I want them to see Christ in me and to desire Him just as much as I do. When I accepted Jesus as my Lord and Savior, it was no longer I who lived but Christ who lives in me. I know the closer I get to God the more people will talk about me and dislike me. It's happening already, when I talk about God I see people smirking with the look of disbelief on their faces. My mother says that I talk about God too much, but I should be talking about Him more. My mom tells me that I'm on fire for the Lord, but it won't last forever. The devil is a liar because I love the Lord with all my heart and soul. I will keep praying and I will keep walking and being obedient to God's will. Sometimes my flesh tries to rise up and cause me to sin but I crucify my flesh daily. I will take up my cross and follow Jesus as I strive to do what is right in God's sight. When satan does try to attack me I still praise God because I know that he has no power over me and cannot harm me. I continuously pray and ask God to give me wisdom and understanding. Sometimes I cry when I think about the things I do because I want to do what is right yet I do what is wrong. The things that the flesh desire is the exact opposite of what God has called me to do. Tomorrow is not promised to me and I just want to move forward. I know that I have to stop gossiping about people and I ask the Lord to help me. I will be mindful of people's feelings and always treat everyone with love. I must forgive myself along with forgiving everyone else as my Father in heaven has forgiven me. I will tell everyone about God and what he has done for me. When I do what is sinful it only angers God and turns my life upside down. I must stop giving in to my sinful desires. I am so grateful to know God and to know that I can always depend on Him. I will be glad and rejoice no matter what the situation is because God is so good. I must be ready at all times for the return of Christ. I will always continue to love the Lord and seek a relationship with Him. I will ask for help when I need it and I will continue to study, pray and meditate on scriptures. I must repent and turn from sin and seek God's face daily. I will always remember that God richly provides me with all that I need. I will always share and be generous to others. I asked God to circumcise my heart by cutting away everything inside of me that's not like Him. There is no reason for me to worry about anything. If I just trust in God, He will carry me through because He loves me so much and He never will leave me. I will live my life in the Spirit and walk by faith and not by sight. I thank God that He has filled me with the Holy Ghost so that I will not believe false teachings. I will always pray to be where God has called me to be. My desire is to be ready to help others at all times. In every situation and circumstance I trust God. When I think I am suffering or when I am going through trials, I remember all that God has brought me through. One of the most wonderful things about God is that He is the same yesterday, today and forever. I've found out that no matter what I do, it's impossible to please some people so I'll focus on pleasing God. I want to live each day as if it were my last. I won't worry about how many days

I have left, but I will make the best out of the time that I do have.

I will praise Him for bringing me out of my troubles. I will continue to pray, fast and study the word of God. As I come closer to God, He will come closer to me. I will keep praying and believing that God will fix the things in my life that seem impossible. He will direct my path.

I was created for God's purpose and I will show my love for Him by working to win souls. I will not hesitate to share my testimony of the greatness of our Lord. I will work diligently not to repeat unkind words or gossip at any time. I will seek God in all that I do and ask Him to show me His will and to strengthen me to do what is right. I will bless the Lord at all times for all that He's done for me. I will keep pouring the word of God into my belly to strengthen my roots. Nothing is more important to me than God. I thank Him for everything He's done. I know I could never repay God for all He's done for me, but I am determined to try. I will seek God's will before I do anything. I'll ask Him to direct my path and this way I won't get lost. I'm a child of God and now I must live and act like who I am. I pray for understanding of the word of God and I will apply the scriptures to my life. I fear the Lord so much and I love Him just as much. I will arm myself with the word of God so that I can withstand the schemes of the devil. Temptation will come but I will submit myself to God, resist the devil and he will flee. I have no cares or worries on earth other than fulfilling God's purpose for my life. I'm so grateful to serve such a mighty God. I thank God that He has given me the grace to endure the tough times that I have seen. Prior to now, I've heard people talk about God every now and then but I didn't know Him for myself. Lord, I thank you that I am safe in your bosom now. I know that there is a God and Christ lives on the inside of me. Through all of my trials and tribulations I never could have made it without Him. I just have to say "thank you" for all you've done for me. Thank you for loving me in spite of all the things I've done. The enemy has tried to set traps for me, but God lifted me out. It seemed like I had fallen into a deep dark pit with no way out. I was so far down looking up and crying out for help and I didn't think anyone could hear me. I thought I would die in that dark place but God was with me even then.

He'll never leave me nor forsake me and when I cried out to him, He brought me out. I thought He couldn't hear me but He hears everything. I let the enemy convince me that I was too far gone to be rescued, but God had a plan for my life. God told me not to worry about anything because He is God and He is in control. I put Him first in my life because of who He is. Now I can see things that I could never see before. He tells me things that will happen before they actually happen. This makes it easier for me to endure. God told me to cast all my cares on Him because He cares for me. I am in this world for God's purpose and my life is not my own. I am the righteousness of God in Christ Jesus and no weapon formed against me can prosper. The scriptures are beginning to come alive in my life. I am a new creature in Christ and all the old has passed away. Behold I am new and I give God all the glory. Everyone in my life has disappointed me or let me down. Lord, I had enough of the false expectations I had of others. I thank you for them being in my life but God it's you that I need.

People were very cruel sometimes by saying things to intentionally hurt and insult me. I already thought I wasn't good enough and I didn't need any help with that. I always felt like I should be doing more to please God because I never want to anger Him. The enemy had convinced me that I was in everyone's way and had no real value or purpose for being here. No matter who I was around I always felt alone and left out. I knew something was wrong with me but I didn't know what it was. It's impossible to fix something when you don't know what's broken. What was I supposed to do besides asking God to fix it? The blood of Jesus covered my sins and the enemy has been defeated. I have the victory over the enemy.

I had a difficult time forgiving myself. In this too I had to seek God. My children and I do talk now more than we used to but not as much as I would like. I used to call my oldest son and for weeks he wouldn't answer the phone or return my calls. Thank God it's not like that anymore and we talk all the time and are quite close. I will concentrate on pleasing God in all I do. People don't forget your past and they never seem to stop reminding you of it. I don't want to think about my past because it makes things difficult for me. It's the enemy trying to keep me from moving forward and being closer to God. I cried so much until I was drained and I just wanted it to stop. I've been deeply hurt from the things that were said to me and about me even although some of it was true. Help me Lord for this is too much for me to bare. God says to cast my burdens on Him and He will sustain me. I wanted to stop crying but I couldn't. I was told that tears are cleansing and in that case I was surely clean by now. Every time I told myself I wouldn't cry I cried anyway. I just couldn't control it. God says that there will always be trials and sorrows in this life but Jesus overcame the world. It seems like I'm the only one going through troubles but no one is exempt from the wilderness. It seemed like instantly God delivered me out of the darkness and into the light.

I thank God for each and every day that He gives me. When I wake up in the mornings I get out of bed because I am excited to live for Christ. Thinking about God makes me happy and now that I have Him, I have everything I need. He is my happiness, my joy, my peace, my provider and my healer. I thought I was having fun living the way the world lives but my life is just now beginning. I am a child of God and He loves me unconditionally. He delivered me and I have to remember that everything doesn't change immediately. Walking with God is a process and I thank Him for leading me all the way through it. When I rededicated my life to the Lord, I knew I would spend it working to please Him. I repented of all my sins, and asked God to cleanse me of all unrighteousness. God looks at the inside and not what's on the outside. He is the only one who knows that I never meant to hurt anyone. I certainly never wanted to disappoint or disobey God. I know that when I repented, God forgave me but I couldn't forgive myself for the things I had done. It was eating away at me on the inside. But then I found out that unforgiveness is a sin too. I just couldn't seem to forgive myself, so I asked God to help me. Sometimes we have to go through things, but we also grow through things. God uses these trials to build our endurance and character. I've had plenty of trouble and sorrows in my life but nothing is too hard for God. No matter how hard I tried I couldn't stop thinking about the past.

I was filled with guilt and shame. The people around me always reminded me of the things I used to do. Some say they need time to trust me because of all I did in the past. The enemy used my family to hurt me the most. He knows how powerful a family is when they come together on one accord. He tries to cause division in families because a house divided cannot stand. I had to choose whether I wanted to please my family or please God. At first I tried to please them but no matter what I did, it wasn't good enough. I kept going to church, praying to God and reading the bible. One day I read that I must love God more than anyone else and this helped me to move on.

I thank God for delivering me from the spirit of addiction. I have to continue to speak this over my life and trust in God because He is good. I tried so many times to stop using on my own but God was waiting for me to submit to Him. I kept telling myself that I wouldn't use anymore but I always did. I was so hard on myself because I thought I should be strong enough to stop on my own.

Every time I relapsed I nosedived into a deep depression and I continued to get high. I felt useless, hopeless and so guilty and ashamed. I had to learn how to pray and how to wait on God to move in my life. I would get so frustrated because I was asking God to help me and I didn't understand why He wasn't. I tried to figure out why God would allow me to keep using drugs even though I didn't want to. People were telling me that I should not keep using while asking God to deliver me. But I couldn't make them understand that I didn't have a choice because the spirit was controlling. I was afraid and I didn't know that I have authority over the power of the enemy. I heard so many speeches about how we have choices in life but it was never my choice to be an addict. I knew that was not what I wanted to do, but I was lost and I needed God in my life.

Living for God is exciting and I can't think of a better feeling than being in His presence. I will walk with Him and be obedient to Him. I will always desire to be in His presence. God knows my heart and I trust in Him completely. I will acknowledge Him in all my ways and He will direct my path. I will come closer to God and He will come closer to me. Lord, I want to hear you clearly as you guide me along the path for which you created me. Lord, I thank you for hearing my prayers. Life is so short, we're here one day and gone the next so I won't spend time worrying. I'll pray about everything, thank God for what He's done and tell Him what I need. Sometimes when I read the bible I still can't make sense out of what I've read, but I keep on reading and hoping that God gives me understanding. I know how much He loves me and wants me to get things right and I will. I thank Him for being so patient with me. I know that if I give in to the desires of my flesh this will separate me from God. I will put God first in everything I do. I don't need to worry about tomorrow because today is hard enough. Lord, I ask you to cleanse me of my old ways and destroy all things inside me that are not like you. My heart's desire is to live according to the will of God. I submit myself to God and resist the devil and he will flee. No matter how others feel about me I know how valuable I am to God. The devil creeps around in the darkness seeking to devour me but the spirit of the Lord is my light and salvation. I will continue to seek ye first the kingdom of God. The bible says to rejoice even in suffering and be patient and wait on the Lord. I will confess and repent of every sin I can think of and those I have forgotten about too. I cannot hold hurt, anger, pain, bitterness and disappointment inside me because this is sin too.

I invited God to go into the secret and hidden places in my heart. I must guard my heart at all times because out of it flow the issues of life. I will keep my eyes on the prize which is the kingdom of heaven. I cannot and will not be side tracked by anything or anyone.

Oh Lord, restore my joy back to me. We are all a part of one body, the body of Christ and all my answers lie in God. I must never be overcome with fear because God has not given me a spirit of fear, but of love, power and a sound mind. No matter what happens in my life, I know God will carry me through it. I know God will never leave me nor forsake me and He knows what's best for me. I will stay focused and listen closely to the instructions of the Lord. I will work day and night to please God and I will stay away from evil. After the storm is over there will be joy. I will remain humble and grateful, thanking God for all He's done. Patience, kindness, love, joy, peace, goodness, faithfulness and self-control; these are the fruits of the spirit. My desire is for them to be seen in everything I do and say. I know I can do it because I can do all things through Christ who strengthens me. I must show love and kindness to all of God's people and never treat anyone differently. God sees all and knows all; therefore, I will do what is right according to His will and His word. When things get tough I will call on the name of the Lord. When I'm overwhelmed I will call on the Lord. Every time the Lord whispers to me with instructions I will be ready. I will be obedient to His every command. I owe God so much and I could never repay Him for all He's done for me. There is no one like God. Who would send their only Son to the earth to suffer and bare our sins? Thank you Jesus for coming to save the world! When I think about Jesus being crucified on the cross to save me, tears begin to stream down my face. I think about how great He is because knew that He would be betrayed by one of His disciples, yet He never treated him any differently. Many of us have rejected Him and yet He still prays and intercedes for us. Jesus suffered so much for us and I am eternally grateful. The bible tells us that we must suffer as Christ suffered. As I face challenges, I am reminded that my suffering is nothing compared to all that Jesus endured for me. This is why I am so eager and enthusiastic to tell everyone about the Good News. I thank God every day for the air that I breathe. I will not look to man for his approval instead, I will trust and depend on God because He is in control and there is no end to His greatness. I will always do the things that God commands me to do and this way I won't be hurt.

God does not lie and He won't leave me and I'll never leave Him.

Today I walk with my head up and a smile on my face. God has delivered me, cleaned me up and set me free from the spirit of addiction. Today I live with an addiction that's different from all the rest. I am addicted to loving, serving and pleasing God. I'm addicted to doing His will. I'm addicted to praising Him for all that He's done for me. Being addicted to God makes me dance, clap and sing praises to Him. This addiction leaves me smiling instead crying. I will rejoice in the Lord at all times. Nothing in this world could ever cause me to turn away from God. The hard thing for me now is when I think I've disappointed God or been disobedient. I make mistakes all the time and the enemy tries to use them to keep me in condemnation. But as I continue to study the word of God, I know there is no condemnation for those who are in Christ Jesus. I still cry a lot but it's no longer because I'm broken, it's because I love the Lord with all my heart and soul. No one knew my story until now, but God told me to stop hiding because He did this for me. I boast only on God because He deserves it. I won't let shame, guilt or fear stop me from talking about the goodness of the Lord. I am so thankful for everything God is doing in my life. I hope that someone hears or sees my story and understands what an awesome God we serve. I went through this to encourage someone else so that they too can be set free. God is the same yesterday, today and forever more. He did it for me and He'll do it for you.